For PAT,

Queen of the Burnsville Buffaloes,
I'll be on your team for as
long as it takes.

Keep the Faith.

Warm regards
and much love,

Jamie

"Bob Stone is an extraordinary human being with a unique approach to conquering cancer. His experience can help so many patients in their battle against this disease. Bob's example has shown us not only how to live with cancer, but how to live.

"Where the Buffaloes Roam: Building A Team for Life's Challenges is a wonderful book that will inspire, support, and comfort cancer patients worldwide. 'The Buffaloes' have recaptured the power and vision of a community where people care deeply for one another. They remind us that we live in a world that is much in need of teams."

—Robert C. Bast, Jr., M.D.
Director, Duke Comprehensive Cancer Center

Where the Buffaloes Roam

Where the Buffaloes Roam

BUILDING A TEAM FOR LIFE'S CHALLENGES

Bob Stone and
Jenny Stone Humphries

ADDISON-WESLEY PUBLISHING COMPANY

Reading, Massachusetts   Menlo Park, California   New York
Don Mills, Ontario   Wokingham, England   Amsterdam   Bonn
Sydney   Singapore   Tokyo   Madrid   San Juan
Paris   Seoul   Milan   Mexico City   Taipei

Library of Congress Cataloging-in-Publication Data

Stone, Bob (Robert Tyler), 1940–
    Where the buffaloes roam : building a team for life's challenges/
Bob Stone and Jenny Stone Humphries.
       p.   cm.
   ISBN 0-201-62641-1
   1. Stone, Bob (Robert Tyler), 1940—Health. 2. Kidneys—Cancer—
Patients—United States—Biography. 3. Cancer-Psychological aspects.
I. Humphries, Jenny Stone. II. Title
362.1'9699'4610092—dc20
RC280.K5S767   1993
[B]   93-15917
                                          CIP

First published in 1993 by Lapidum Press

Jacket design by Jean Seal

1 2 3 4 5 6 7 8 9-MA-96959493
First printing, July 1993

DEDICATION

I have been on Life's journey for fifty-two years and the thing that makes it interesting are the people a loving God places in my path. He lets me know He's there by sending me hands-on help when I need it most.

When I was diagnosed with an incurable type of cancer, Lloyd Peterson, my doctor-friend, knew how to communicate the bad news and, at the same time, give me hope—a wonderful gift for a healer. The hugs and support that Patsy and Frank Kendall gave us that first night were a great comfort. My prayer group buddies of thirteen years, Vic Cochran, David Grimes, and Larry Sitton were waiting to help me around the next bend. They still are. Jerry Shelter was not only our pastor but the friend who introduced me to the books of Bernie Siegel, Norman Cousins, and Deepak Chopra.

I am indebted to my parents for their love and foundation in faith—my mother's humor and my father's determination. Both must be in the gene pool because Cousin Jenny, with her keen sense of humor and great talent, wrote that first letter which let me know there could be joy in the moment. Then another cousin, Bill Stone, was at my side in a matter of hours, helping put my legal affairs in battle-ready order for what lay ahead.

What lay ahead was the Duke Comprehensive Cancer Center. Drs. Bob Bast and Phil Walther gave me the opportunity to prove that medical technology, the nursing staff on the Jordan Ward, and a responsive immune system can beat the odds.

My own two, Tyler and Marion, found the parent-child roles reversed and became sensitive and stalwart caregivers. I learned a lot from them. My big sister, Martha, let me know each and every day for seven months by phone, card, letter and dire threat that giving up was not an option. Getting well seemed the course of least resistance.

I am grateful to the Buffaloes—friends, classmates, neighbors, church members, business clients—that signed on to become Undefeatable Champs. I have been strengthened by the cancer patients and their families Genie and I have met over the last two years. I am constantly renewed and inspired by their courage and grace. I am proud to be on *their* team.

Life is richer when it is shared and I've done some world-class sharing with a young woman who thirty years ago, on this very day, said she would love me in sickness and in health and meant every word—my lovely Genie.

How do I say thank you? This book is a beginning.

Bob Stone
July 14, 1992

FOREWORD

This is the story of a team, a team that outgrew its original franchise, a team that wouldn't quit, wouldn't say die. A team that said No to terminal cancer, No to the narrowing of life's options, and went on to carry the guy who brought them together to a quantum victory over cancer.

"I called us the Buffaloes," said Bob Stone. "The buffalo— an endangered species, a dying breed making its comeback now. It seemed to fit!" Bob Stone and his team of Buffaloes are taking their challenges untamed and on the hoof. In this world of broken relationships, litigious and fractious living, ties that rarely bind, the go-for-broke Buffaloes have found the critical mass of family and friends expanding. They have found a richness in their lives that can be translated to others. "Even if I hadn't beaten cancer," Bob says with an easy grin, "the quality of life for both me and my family would have been so much better because of having a team like the Buffaloes behind us. We are all terminal. We all die some time, whether it's in a week or a month or a lifetime from now. What matters is how we live the life we have. I found that win or lose with my cancer, I still won. I won by finding greater closeness with long-time friends, by the excitement of reaching out to total strangers, by the astonishing way the network spun out, faster and farther than I could ever have imagined."

Bob's a great teacher, he's a sage, a guru...People will flock to him to learn how do you deal with adversity, how do you find joy in this moment? Bernie Siegel, M.D., author of *Love, Medicine and Miracles.*

WHERE THE BUFFALOES ROAM

Bernie Siegel is right! Bob Stone and his team have found joy in the moment. The Buffaloes are proof that people are weary of watching life unreel frame by frame in a sitcom. They are tired of being mere onlookers; they want to be participants in this adventure of Life!

Bob has told the team's story on the *CBS This Morning* Show. Groups across the country have been inspired by it. Those who joined Bob's team find themselves reaching out to others, inspiring new teams, new dreams. Bob Stone learned that life is not a death-defying solo act but a team effort.

Let's see how this preacher's kid, Everybody's Best Newsboy, a guy who still believes his breakfast cereal is shot from guns, put together his own world class challenge team.

What the Buffaloes discovered can be applied not just to those battling, or to those supporting someone battling, a serious illness, but to others as well. It is for this year's college senior who wants to stay bonded to his buddies, to the environmentalist who wants to save the South American rain forests, to the activist who hears a call to do something about AIDS. To all who need encouragement to keep the dream alive.

At last count, more than five hundred three-button-suit types, closet screen writers, club ladies, bag ladies, soul mates, play mates—even a world-renowned humanitarian—call themselves Buffaloes. They are all a part of Bob's story—no, the Buffaloes are not a *part* of Bob's story. They *are* his story.

Jenny Stone Humphries

ACKNOWLEDGEMENTS

To Letitia Sweitzer for her friendship. It takes a writer to know a writer. And to my pastor Dr. James E. Long, Jr. for his teaching and a great Albert Schweitzer quotation. And to Melanie Smallie of Bookmark for making a book seem easy.

And to my rambunctious, audacious teammates, the Buffaloes, for their wonderful letters and encouragement. They wrote our book for us.

To our families who showed us the way to go and gave us what we needed to get there.

And, most especially, to my own team:

> Stan
> Sally
> Stanley Bradford
> and my mother, Virginia Stone

> Jenny Stone Humphries

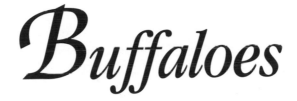

Where the Buffaloes Roam

PROLOGUE

The sun had caught fire just over the ridge of mountains beyond our bedroom window. I could smell coffee and something even better--Genie's homemade cinnamon bread. A Brandenburg concerto was spinning out from the tape deck downstairs, lending an elegant structure to the morning. I highly recommend Bach as an indispensable adjunct to your self-realization and positive thinking program. These heavy metal guys can't even get in Bach's game.

The sun was burning off the early morning haze. I could see Grandfather Mountain in the distance. They tell us the largest crystal formation in the country is right on top of that mountain. A mountain top of pure crystal!

Maggie, our golden retriever, bolted up the stairs and into the bedroom and began tugging at the bedcovers. We mountain folk get up early and slug-a-beds are not tolerated.

After coffee and Bach, I launched myself into a new day. Bob Macauley, founder of AmeriCares, a world-wide humanitarian organization, had asked me to call Egil Hagen of Oslo, Norway.

Egil Hagen. Even the man's name carried the lofty sound of an eagle's wings. Egil Hagen, the renowned humanitarian who had almost single-handedly saved the lives of hundreds of thousands of starving human beings in the famine-devastated Sudan, a genius who had a global vision for this sundered, suffering world and a heart to go with it, had cancer.

Egil Hagen and his doctors in Norway had heard of promising trial therapy being conducted in this country, and now he was seeking information and encouragement from a survivor of the IL-2 Plus LAK campaigns.

1

I could hear the strength in Dounia Hagen's voice as she told me of Egil's condition. "My husband has made his decision. He will fight this cancer he has—what do you think?"

I certainly didn't have to tell Egil Hagen how precious the gift of life was. Here was a man who was obviously ready to tackle another challenge as big as the Sudan.

"Sure, he should fight it! I think that's exactly what he should do, Dounia!"

I looked down and Maggie was on her haunches, assuming her ready-to-counsel-position. She'd heard my story before. Maggie had heard more than her share of my stories. "Dounia," I said, "Let me tell you about some of the things I've found to be helpful—" Maggie's tail began to thump rhythmically. "What you need to do is get yourself a team," I said. Now Maggie was beating a happy cadence. Maggie knew about teams.

ONE

Hardball at Handball

Life not only seemed good, it *was* good. I was one lucky guy and I knew it. I headed my own benefit planning firm, took an active part in church, the community, and was an active alum at my alma mater, Davidson College. My wife Genie and I had invested twenty-nine years in one marriage—*that* spells commitment. Our two kids, Tyler and Marion, were out on their own now and showing a lot of promise, as they say in my part of piedmont North Carolina. My sister Martha claims that I'm the kind of guy who just *looks* like everybody's brother. I offer that as a testimonial.

The only documented case of substance abuse in the family was when Chris, our wild-at-heart Lab, OD-ed on a five-pound sack of penny candy. My doctor certainly would have agreed that physically, Bob Stone was in enviable shape for a guy who had just turned fifty.

Then an afternoon of hard ball on the handball court and an ominous warning signal put me across the desk from my doctor friend, changing not only the ground rules Bob Stone played by, but the game itself.

I'd been working non-stop getting ready for a big presentation coming up. By Thursday afternoon the team at the office had things in good shape. I had nothing more pressing on my mind than working off some of the day's load of stress with a game of handball. I finished my game, showered and dressed. I basked in that feeling of well-being you get after a great workout. I could hold my own at handball. I jogged, biked, watched my weight. I'd recently passed an intensive insurance physical that left no Stone unturned—not this one anyway.

I shoved my gear in my gym bag and headed home. After dinner Genie had promised to show me the plans for the Charleston garden she was putting in back of our house in Greensboro. There were enough bricks stacked in our backyard to construct our own Appian Way. I headed home to admire Genie's pile of brick. I felt great!

At my office the next morning I took a break and ducked into the men's room. There was blood in my urine. That got my attention in a hurry. An ominous alarm clanged in my head, slamming into my ready alert system like that hard rubber ball coming off the handball court straight at me. I knew it was bad.

I couldn't get to a telephone fast enough. "Come on in now" my friend, Lloyd, who is a urologist, urged. I didn't need any urging, let me tell you.

From that point on things shifted into fast forward. My friend in the white coat was guarded. "Hematuria, blood in the urine, not good," he scolded. "Do you have to play handball like the Terminator? How many miles are you running these days? Lloyd was a marathon runner and had a deadly backhand on the tennis court. He'd get me back in playing shape. "Let's do a sonargram and take some X-rays."

Suddenly I began to pick up disturbing signals while on the table. Warning flags go up like storm flags being hoisted off the Outer Banks—the way Lloyd and the technician looked at each other, the way they tried so hard to keep things calm. It was like looking on while they loaded the last life boat on the Titanic, pretending this was a drill instead of the real thing.

"Bob, you've got a large tumor on that left kidney," Lloyd's face was grave, as he seated himself across the desk from me in his office. "It's got to come out right away, that much we know. It's more than likely cancerous. I'll schedule you for surgery next week. We'll know more Monday when we do the CAT scan and the other tests."

Cancer was no stranger to our family. But tragically, the same can be said for most of our homes across this nation. No one is untouched by the disease. The stats say one million people will hear the word "cancer" from their doctors this year. And half of them will die from it. Most of us have more than a casual brush with the disease.

What to this day strikes me as unbelievable was my own reaction. I wasn't angry, I wasn't scared, I wasn't bitter. I just wanted to get on with the program. I know now that my reaction was my way of approaching something too enormous to take in. If my mind had been a computer it would have typed out: internal system failure. Mentally I was doing the only thing I knew to do, taking one step at time; I refused to even think of telling Genie until I got the results of the CAT scan and other tests back. I wanted more information, the advice of specialists, resource people. I had friends in the Duke University medical community. Genie and I served on the Citizens Advisory Committee for the Duke Comprehensive Cancer Center and helped with their fund-raisers.

A few blocks away, my minister at First Presbyterian was in his study preparing his Sunday sermon. I considered calling my Monday morning irregulars—Vic, Larry, and David, the three guys who have shared my life and my prayers for the last thirteen years. For this son of a Presbyterian minister, prayer was simply a way of keeping God current.

That night I had the Daddy of all nightmares. It was King, Spielberg, and Kafka all rolled into one midnight horror show. In my dream, a hideous praying mantis-like creature was locked inside a kidney-shaped prison chamber, frantically clawing, thrashing and fighting to get out. I woke up doing some powerful thrashing myself. It certainly made me wonder if the body doesn't have its own graphic way of telling you what is wrong...and where. What my own body was telling me was there was a monster loose and it was trying to kill me.

The Motion Picture Academy gave an Academy Award to

5

Jessica Tandy and Morgan Freeman for "Driving Miss Daisy" but it should have been Bob Stone's for his role in "No Way Out." Genie and I went to a friend's home for dinner, Genie blessedly unaware of my red alert. You'd think I had the world by the string instead of dangling by the frailest shred of one.

All during those hours over that weekend I cannot honestly say I was obsessed with the thought of dying. It wasn't the thought of death that washed over me again and again that weekend but something else entirely—the bittersweet sadness of goodbye. I wondered, was this what it was like for my sister Mary when she sat in her doctor's office at Emory University Hospital, the ghostly reverse image her own rib cage looming out at her? Did she experience this same sharp sweet feeling that caught in her chest, both loving and hating this world so much in a single heart-stopping moment?

Mary's doctors gave her nine months. I think Mary accepted that calendar they handed her and began to mark off the days. When her nine months were up, Mary died. Quietly, bravely, and totally without hope. That was the worst part—not giving her the slightest shred of hope to hang on to.

TWO

Wake-Up Call

The CAT scans on Monday were grim. The report read:

Chest CT showed 4-5 small scattered lesions, undoubtedly metastatic tumor. Liver on CT scan showed several small lesions which could be either cyst or metastatic disease. Looks like the proximal renal vein had tumor in it. Spleen may also be invaded locally.

This is not what Bob Stone wants to hear. I want to hear that the excellent care I've taken of myself has paid off, that I'm a winner, a perfect specimen who will more than likely be fly-fishing at ninety. Handball is simply not my sport.

The complete readings and test results were no better. The cancer had spread to my lymph glands, spleen, lungs, and possibly my liver.

It was obvious that a quick radical nephrectomy couldn't begin to handle this problem. I needed an industrial-strength miracle. My mind was sweeping ahead, clicking off the information the doctor gave me.

Metastatic kidney cancer is extremely resistent to standard treatment used for other cancers. Chemotherapy and radiation have little effect. Researchers have tried every new therapy of promise over the last thirty years with little results. Only a victim of malignant melanoma can claim the same dismal prospects.

Obviously racking his brain for something hopeful, my doctor suggested I might possibly fit the profile at the National Cancer Institute. Dr. Steven Rosenberg at NCI had developed an approach administering Interleukin-2, (IL-2). IL-2 is a hormone released by the T lymphocyte white cells in the immune system which stimulates production of Lymphokine-Activated Killer cells (LAK cells). These LAK cells are cancer killers; they go on a search and destroy mission, killing tumor cells and reducing the size of tumors.

I walked out of my urologist's office into a brilliant February afternoon. The sun was shining, the air was winter cool on my face, a few blades of grass struggled up from a crack in the sidewalk, my car was waiting at the curb, with time still on the meter. Everything was just as I'd left it two hours ago, except for one thing. I was dying.

I understood exactly what a "worst-case scenario" was. I was it. When it came to a quick fix for my cancer, I was a day late and a dollar short.

Telling my wife Genie was the toughest thing I've ever had to do. For her it was the same bad dream happening all over again. Genie had lost her mother to cancer. They were very close. She still can't talk about her mother without tears. And now it was me. I had always been a caregiver in the family, the big guy who can make anything all right—anything, except renal cell carcinoma.

Anyone who knows me will tell you I'm not a drinking man, not this preacher's boy—maybe an occasional glass of wine with dinner but that's it. The weekend I was keeping my cancer all to myself, I took a drink to help me get to sleep that night. I had some fine aged bourbon—not the back-of-the-closet kind you usually find around my house—but something rare a client had given me for Christmas. I fixed myself a pretty stiff drink. The next evening I fixed both Genie and me a drink. Genie eyed me warily and shot me an "I'm no party pooper" look. Monday evening, after the CAT scans, I steeled myself for the ordeal of telling Genie. Again, I mixed the two of us a drink. Genie was openly aghast. "What's going on here, Bob?" she asked.

All the bourbon in the world wouldn't make what I had to tell her any easier. "Genie, after my handball game the other day I passed some blood in my urine. I trotted right over to Lloyd's office to check it out. Genie, it's real bad. Renal cell carcinoma. Cancer of the kidney."

Have you ever had the feeling that two hearts have suddenly stopped their beating at the same instant? I'll never forget the look on Genie's face. Genie *knew* Cancer; she knew what it meant better than I did. As I told her exactly what the scan had shown, I could see her visibly slipping into deep shock. It was like helplessly watching a loved one go down in icy water. She was shivering, shaking uncontrollably. Genie's reaction made my condition far more real than the X-rays or Lloyd's written report.

Fortunately Genie and I have a friend who's a psychotherapist. Patsy was "a friend indeed to a friend in need" that night. Genie and I drove over to her house and Patsy helped us talk it out together so we could begin to deal with it.

After Genie, there was still Marion and Tyler and my sister Martha to tell, plus Genie's family, as close to me as my own. It was rough sledding for a few days.

Genie called her brother Tom and asked him to break the news to their dad. Then Genie drove with me to Charlotte to tell my sister. Martha's son Johnny booked the next flight out to Montana to tell our daughter Marion, who was in an outdoor leadership program. I told Tyler myself, father to son. And each time there was a fresh raw pain and the grief of having to pass it on to those I loved. But through this searing catharsis, I was forced to come to grips with my own death. I felt its impact each time I shared my tears, my disbelief, my *mortality* with those I loved.

I realize now that it was in that sharing, that telling, that I began to sense the tremendous value of family and support of a group of human beings who care about you. I hadn't begun to think of that group as a team yet but that would come later.

I called my pastor at First Presbyterian and then the news was out. You just can't slam the door shut against yourself and the world out there.

No one can tell you how to face your own death. I was beginning to realize that the reason I hadn't been obsessed with the thought of my own death after Lloyd told me about the CAT scans was simple. I didn't know how to die. I knew how to live. I knew how to start a business, how to check the oil in my car, how to play handball—but dying. Dying was not a learned skill, it was something that happened. Now I know that dying *is* a learned skill and, while some are better at it than others, it is still mandatory for each of us. The problem is, that as human beings, we simply don't think about *not* being. That's the way we are programmed. Sure, we buy insurance, draw up a will, name beneficiaries, but that's for What If. We all feel we are forever. We keep count of those fat grams and shift into aerobic gear several times a week because we want to be healthy while we're marching to Forever.

But after the doctors had their say, it became very necessary for me to accept and come to grips with the reality of death. You have to get comfortable with your own mortality before others can be comfortable enough with you to help and support you.

How could I free all of my energy to the healing process, if I were crippled by the possibility of What-If-I-Don't-Make-It? It is absolutely essential to consider the possibility of death, plan for it, even grieve over it. Only then are you able to muster the spiritual resources you need to get on with the program.

For all of us, there is the big D to get around. Death. Dying. Okay, I kept asking myself, what if I give my all and *still* don't make it? One thing was for sure. If I *didn't* give my all, I certainly wouldn't have a chance of making it. If the worst happened, I would still meet death with more peace of mind knowing I had pulled out all the stops and given it my best.

For many of us Death is that mysterious Dark Continent we studied in our geography book as kids. It had the world's longest river, crocodiles, head hunters, fever, bizarre rituals, strange flora and fauna. The unknown of death can be just as scary for us as that mysterious continent in the geography book.

So much has been written about this great unknown of death. Kubler-Ross and many others have made a study of death and dying. Evidence suggests that dying isn't a hard thing to do. I agree. And now, I speak with some experience.

But, for me, it is Dr. Lewis Thomas in *The Medusa and the Snail* and Timothy Ferris' *Coming of Age in the Milky Way and The Mind's Sky: Human Intelligence in a Cosmic Context* that gives a sense of both the harmonious mystery and adventure of death. Dr. Ferris writes of the transcendent joy and ecstasy that accompanies the experience. "We speak of death as the king of terrors, yet how rarely the act of dying appears to be painful." writes Dr. Ferris. He goes on to say that Lewis Thomas reported that in all his medical experience he had only encountered one incidence of painful death—a case of rabies.

Dr. Ferris suggests that when we have exhausted all medical avenues that our own survival mechanism becomes a fail-safe device that kicks in and lifts us out of distress. Ferris proposes that death is not oblivion but a cosmological event!

So that fearful Dark Continent we approach with such trepidation and terror may actually be our own excellent adventure. And when you believe in life after life, then we truly become explorers of the cosmic universe, with Heaven our tent and Eternity our map.

But I was not quite ready to sign up for that final exploration. I had not yet exhausted all avenues of survival. I had not blown the hatch on Life. Right here seemed good enough for me!

I was like the fellow caught between a rock and a hard place at one of those old fashioned revival meetings we have in the rural churches in the South. The preacher had put everything he had into his sermon. He was drafting like Richard Petty behind a full hour of brimstone and redemption. "All right, good people," he exhorted, "Everyone who wants to be with your Lord in Heaven, raise your hand." Hands shot up all over the fevered congregation. His audience was panting for salvation. All except this one fellow who appeared to be a fence-straddler. "Let me see those hands again," the preacher badgered. All hands went up for a second time except for our taciturn fellow in the back. The preacher just couldn't stand it. He wanted one hundred and ten percent.

"Brother," he said, daring to single the guy out, "Aren't you a believer?"

"I am."

"Brother, don't you want to spend Eternity with your Lord in Heaven?"

"I do."

"Then why didn't you raise your hand?"

The man was obviously a little chary about the whole idea. "I thought you were getting a load up to go right *now!*"

And that was me. I wasn't ready yet to sign up for the next bus load going to Eternity.

THREE

A Call To Arms

After I had hand wrestled with Mortality for a week, I got with the program and checked out my reading list for Cancer Lit 101. I buried myself in books, tapes, and articles. And out of that information overload I found two great guys who were ultimately to change my life far more than the cancer in my left kidney—Bernie Siegel and Norman Cousins. In reading *Anatomy of An Illness, Head First: The Biology of Hope,* and *Love, Medicine and Miracles,* I saw what doctors seem reluctant to recognize. ME. What About Me? What part does Me play in all this? Mr. Cousins and Mr. Siegel introduced Bob Stone to what I've dubbed the Me Factor, the capability we all possess to aid in our own healing. A factor which is different for every individual, a variable—even more interesting, an unknown quantity.

Scientists call this psychoneuroimmunology. It's a mouthful to learn to say, but learn it anyway! This is going to be the buzz word of the coming decade. Psychoneuroimmunology is the science which studies the effect of the mind on the body. The mind-body connection. The ME factor. Cousins and Siegel told me why I wasn't ready to be planted in a hole with a rose bush over my feet. They gave a guy hope.

Suddenly I was more than a statistic or a dreary actuarial write-off, I was the wild card, the no-trump. I had weight, I had heft, I had a position in this high stakes game of my own life and death.

13

I balked and refused to be led gently into that good night where a prudent Calvinist updates his will, buys his wife something that will last, and takes off on a thrifty vacation to Myrtle Beach.

This is not to say I failed to fully appreciate my situation. I understood a system failure, in my business or in my body. The immune system is a complex computer programmed to override most failures in the system. But as awesome as the immune system is, it can fail. That same system is prey to an irresponsible hacker, breaking into an efficiently running program, breaching all safeguards, planting bugs, glitches, infecting the system with mysterious viruses which cause the body to turn on itself and become a Doomsday machine, throwing out cancer cells faster than the immune system's pacman can gobble them up.

But my urologist had given me a glimpse of hope in the program he had told me about at the National Cancer Institute. I was more determined than ever to get accepted into the program. Put in realtor's jargon, I was highly motivated. The National Cancer Institute and Dr. Steven Rosenberg were onto something promising with this IL-2 Plus LAK. To be sure it was a distant hope I glimpsed, but I pursued it. It was not only my best hope, it seemed absolutely my only hope.

I went on the attack.

The National Cancer Institute was a hard sell. It was a daunting place—the Pentagon of modern medicine, the cutting edge of our most advanced research. A compass would have come in handy to find my way in a wilderness of hallways, offices, waiting rooms.

I was milling around in this medical morass when I ran into two other lonely pilgrims. They were just kids, one twelve, the other a couple of years older. They were alone. And like three heifers cut from the herd we stuck together. We made small talk, shared cookies and juice. I wondered who left these kids to make their own way through this labyrinth. Where were their people?

Cancer can be a lonely business. I will never forget how lonely. Waiting outside Admissions with those two sick kids in a vast place like NCI, it was easy to understand how a person could simply shut down, crawl into himself, and say, this is too big, too hard, too lonely, too dicey. You wait to be called, you wait to be treated, you wait to hear the results. That's when I began to think about how I could overcome the isolation that is a part of serious illness.

Subconsciously I was already thinking *team* to back me in the biggest challenge of my life. Finding camaraderie with those two young men helped relieve the terror and boredom of those hours and hours of waiting. Why not a team? It seemed a natural. That's the way I've learned to run my business, and the projects I've been asked to head, like the Davidson Annual Fund and the Child Care Ministry. I learned early on that I'm no genius, so I'm savvy enough to pick some solid folks to line up with me. If I have a talent it's learning how to put people together and get them working as a team. Benefit packages get put together and sold by the team concept. Genie and I were a team from the word Go; with the kids we had another team. Giving every guy plenty of room to do what he does best is what I believe in.

When I was finally called into the Admissions office at NCI, I wasted no time shifting into the famed Carolina full court press. "I'm going to be the most fun guy you've ever had at NCI," I told them. "We're all going to learn a lot together." I was lucky I wasn't arrested and booked for Assault with a Deadly Disease.

If the counselor had so much as dropped an Admit slip on the floor, I would have tap danced and played a little music on my pocket comb. But Admissions was unimpressed. They put me and my renal cells on Hold. They asked for more lab tests, an additional stress test because my EKG revealed Wolff-Parkinson-White syndrome, a fluky heart irregularity that could cause a valve to act up. NCI would let me know. I was in limbo. But at least I was getting a very positive reading that here at NCI someone was doing more about Cancer than offering a dot-to-dot Last Will & Testament.

I was flying home on a commuter hop, after a long day of playing Hurry And Wait with the medical protocol when I got the idea that was to customize my communications network. The little

15

commuter plane was bucking rough head winds. I was buckled in my seat, thinking about that logjam of messages that would be waiting for me on my answering machine. It was impossible to keep on top of all the calls, but anyone who took the time to telephone certainly deserved more than a impersonal recording machine.

I suddenly noticed the pilot was receiving constant updates on a twenty-four hour weather channel. Great idea! Why not broadcast up-to-date advisories on my status, day by day, for friends who called? I could record the message myself. When the weather got too rough for me to handle, Genie could give my weather report: "Good Morning, you have reached your 24-hour Stone Weather Station! Sunny skies and optimum temperatures over DC today. Outlook is promising for the week ahead." What better way to let friends know how things were going?

I had been advised to line up an oncologist to provide information and to answer our questions. Genie made the appointment for us. When searching questions were asked on the telephone about our financial responsibility and insurance coverage we became uneasy. The doctor's waiting room was as impersonal and cold as the questions put to us. "I understand you're a realist, Mr. Stone", the doctor said, brusquely pinning my X-rays in the viewing box. The storm warnings went up again as I realized with a sinking feeling that this doctor's "realism" was a synonym for doom.

It was true that not much good could be said about those X-rays in the viewer but there was still the Me factor. "How do you feel about visualization techniques?" I asked Doctor Doom. A curt shrug dismissed my question. "Read *Head First* or any of the Bernie Siegel books?" I plodded doggedly ahead. That loosed a diatribe of anger and negativity. Genie and I exited in a powerful hurry and headed for the nearest bomb shelter.

I'm sure that doctor, like many, can point with justifiable pride to patients he has helped, but in my own mind he is a perfect example of what my sister Mary encountered, downside medicine. A caregiver who consciously or unconsciously transmits

16

negative signals to his patients; there's a word for it— off-putting.

In my mind I pushed Rewind and ran the visit through again —this time the way I'd have handled the interview. "Bob, I understand you're a realist. The stats on renal cell carcinoma look terrible." (He tells me how terrible.) "But there's always that exceptional patient. I believe you can be one of them, Bob. Let me tell you how I would like to approach the problem. Let me tell you what I hope we can do working together."

There, that's a much better run-through, isn't it? I admit it—when it comes to hope, I buy the whole nine yards.

Life is not unlike one of the benefit policies my company offers. Life has to be fully vested to be worth anything. We have to put all the hope, heart, intelligence, and love we have or can borrow into life, in order to have something to cash in when we need it.

The history of Man has been marked by brave and restless migrations across the continents in search of sanctuary. And hope. What marks us as a higher species is the hope which informs our life and dreams, even in our most desperate circumstance.

Hope is the radioactive material of the human spirit. It burns through mountains of despair, the sealed containers of indifference, the buried nuclear waste of humanity. Hope is our history, our legacy, our gift. And I believe that the absence of hope was as much responsible for my sister's death as lung cancer.

Days later word came down from NCI. I was in! I was ecstatic. I would have this cancer thing licked in short order with the front line at NCI backing me up.

Then twenty-four hours before I was to check into the hospital, I got a phone call. Sorry, the folks at NCI said, we've just given your test results another thorough reading and our cardiologist is concerned that the Wolff-Parkinson-White syndrome will cause a problem. In all good conscience we can't give you the go-ahead.

I had been cut from the program. My world suddenly spun out from under me for the second time. My bag was packed, airline tickets were laid out on the hall table. NCI, which had seemed so close, might as well be another planet away.

The days that followed my turndown were agonizing. Anxiety, shock, helplessness proliferated in the face of a medical protocol that wouldn't give. Numbly, I tried to regroup and remake shattered plans. New decisions had to be made. Where to go for help? The clock was ticking. And the cancer in my body was continuing to grow unchallenged.

I was learning a hard lesson. I would have liked nothing more than to shove my cancerous kidney with its buckshot of tumors over to NCI and say, "Here guys, take care of this." But first, last, and always, you alone have control of your illness and you have to find your own miracles. You can't depend wholly on someone else; your number one resource is what you can put together for yourself. NCI was a valuable but tough learning experience.

My friends in the Duke medical community had been among the first to offer support. Bob Bast, Director of the Duke Comprehensive Cancer Center, was a good friend. Now Bob charged into the breach left by NCI.

"You need to think about the Duke Comprehensive Cancer Center," Bob Bast told me. "Let me make a few calls and talk to some of our people. You may fit our protocol here. Let's see what we can do."

I was impressed with the program at Duke—that's why Genie and I had helped with their activities. I knew the people there had a very human, holistic approach to dealing with the disease. And they had something else. The Duke Comprehensive Cancer Center was conducting trials with IL-2 Plus LAK.

My dad taught me to believe that for every door that is slammed in your face, another is opened for you. I was, and am to this day, convinced that the best thing I ever did was walk through the door they opened for me at the Duke Comprehensive Cancer Center. That turndown at NCI made me even more determined to beat this cancer and the folks at Duke were going to help me do it!

FOUR

Field Marshall to the Rescue

In the midst of all this turmoil, the morning mail brought a letter from my first cousin, Jenny Stone Humphries. She was my childhood cohort and is now a writer. And as if one of Jenny wasn't enough they cloned her! Jenny and her twin sister, Betty, spent two weeks with my two sisters and me each summer of our growing-up years. We plotted insurrection, waged Monopoly wars, and fought the boredom of quarantines imposed by outbreaks of polio. Jenny seemed to know my genes the way she knew the terrain of our childhood. Her letter shouted encouragement all the way from Georgia to the Carolinas:

> *We have really been rocked by what has happened, as I am sure you have been too, in spades. We do not accept this! I am sorry that you are being deluged with phone calls from all of us who feel the same way. This is what you get for leading a good upright life—if you were a scum-bag nobody would care. And we do.*
>
> *...And I know that same fellow who sold the most newspaper subscriptions and won a bike is going to win again.*
>
> *I leave you with Field Marshall Foch's pithy*

communication from the front during The Great War:

> *My center is giving way, my right is in retreat. Situation is excellent. I am attacking.*

Guess who won? You better believe it!

> *Love, Jenny*

Where did the inspiration for that off-the-wall challenge come from? "Actually I swiped that Field Marshall Foch quote from something I had read in Mother Jones," Jenny told me later. But it was definitely a booster shot of vim and vinegar for this fellow. I rushed out of my office, waving the letter like a battle flag. I read it aloud to my staff. We cheered, whooped, applauded! Our laughter that day told me there could be some fun along with the grimness of disease.

I began outlining my strategy for the season ahead. I made a list of my personal priorities to keep me focused:

A positive mental attitude—Full speed ahead and damn the torpedoes—was my highest priority. You have to focus on yourself and your doctors, rather than the odds which are against you. I quite simply could not afford to whine over spilled milk at NCI. I had to believe that the doctors at Duke could do the job for me, and do it better than anyone else.

The support of family—After God, my family has been as solid and enduring as the Carolina Blue Ridge in my life. In this day of fractured marriages, sundered lives, broken relationships, unfinished agendas, I recognized that I really have something going for me in my twenty-nine years with Genie and the family.

A strong spiritual belief—My dad and mother had given me a simple religious faith that told me *nothing* was impossible with God on your side. I don't have to sift through a myriad of possibilities or entities or incarnations. This Jesus who lived in an underdeveloped country called Galilee sold me on the benefit package He put together. And for me, His package was a big positive.

Spiritual Beliefs are an important part of living a full and abundant life. They are of mega importance in developing and maintaining a positive mental outlook. If there is nothing beyond ourselves, if what life is about is simply gratifying our own whims and needs, then we are locked into a circular, closed kind of existence, and one about as interesting as a can of peas. There has to be an endgame, a point to all this loving and living we do. There has to be something outside the selfishness of self.

You can pick up any alternative newspaper or weekend guide and see hundreds of self-help and support groups from Creative Divorce to How to Tap Your Inner Power. They tell us how to become more articulate, more caring, more responsive. What they don't say is what are we to do with this finer, nobler, better creature? What are we to do with Self?

Many of us end up so bewildered by our many options that we end up doing nothing. We stall out. I'm no preacher and I'm not out to strong arm anyone, but if you're looking for a personal recommendation, I have one for you. Try God.

Family and friends were quick to respond as news of my illness spread. My cousin, Bill, who is an attorney, called and offered not only encouragement but much needed hands-on help. Papers, policies, and business affairs were put in battle-ready order. (That comes under the category of addressing the big bad D word.) Attorneys and financial managers take note.

Neighbors called and left messages. They sent notes, flowers, casseroles, and my favorite chocolate chip cookies. Everyone wanted to help. *So why not let them?*

Standing in my kitchen one afternoon, wallowing in this wonderful glut of caring, my thoughts over these past days began to crystallize. Why *not* pull this caring and concern into something that could become a sustaining *life* force instead of a death vigil? Was it possible that caring, concern, and friendship could produce its own healing energy which could then be transmitted to another person? My reading for Cancer Lit 101 certainly suggested that the answer was Yes. I still had some control over what was happening to me. Okay, that meant I could *choose* those I wanted to share my

21

cancer with. Make sense?

I lifted the cover on a tempting casserole. I was staggered by the gifts of food, the stacks of cards and letters—all the evidence of caring. Friends were great! My spirits lifted. I sure could have used this kind of positive reinforcement at NCI. I suddenly realized that I needed far more than a casserole. I needed the friends who made these casseroles—needed their physical presence, prayers and concern, support. I needed friends to bear with me and my family during this crisis. Where were they when I was holding down that bench in the hall at NCI? Where were *my* people when I stormed out of the office of Doctor Doom? WHERE WAS MY TEAM WHEN I NEEDED THEM?

I decided right then and there to build myself a franchise. I decided to put together a team to go all the way with me—and I meant exactly that—*all the way*. My mind was hurtling ahead. I'd need help running this team. A coach and general manager. Genie won the nod for Coach; it's a role she's played on field and off, under sunny skies or in a downpour—like now. As for GM, I already had the best there is, the God of my fathers. My God too.

Bob Stone was ready to charge onto the field. I was going to get myself a team! The team from nowhere, the team from somewhere—but *where*? My family headed my list, of course. But there were others. I looked at the kitchen counters sagging under the evidence of caring. *Here* was my team, already in place, just waiting for me. What about my friends at Davidson, that football powerhouse of the much feared Colonial conference? *Here* was my team. What about friends in our church, that stronghold of faith, hope and love. *Here* was my team. Messages waited on the answering machine from our study group of couples from Northwestern Mutual. *Here* was my team. Astonished, I discovered I already had a team! All it needed was some organizational skills. Before the afternoon was over, I had a roster of more than a hundred individuals. A hundred individuals who just might possibly be weary of watching sitcoms; people who might be willing, even eager, to get off the bench and be a participant in this very real cliff hanger I had going.

I got excited thinking about that life force out there just waiting to be tapped. But in order to tap into it I would need to take that first step to let people know what was going on in my life. The second step was to let friends know I wanted their help, their prayers, their support. The third step was to tell them *specifically* how they could help.

I hated the idea of a form letter but logistically there was no way around it. But even a form letter would be welcomed if you knew it had something special in it for just you. I resolved that come C-cells or high water, either Genie or I, or both of us, would jot a personal note on each letter sent out.

I drafted a letter, including cousin Jenny's letter with the Field Marshall Foch quote for good measure.

March 16, 1990

Dear Family and Friends,

> *I received the letter on the previous page from my cousin one week after getting my major "wake-up call", and I laugh every time I read the last paragraph. It describes very well the attitude of the Stone camp. We are attacking—and each of you is helping us in this battle more than you know. My parents, my grandparents, and my Sunday School teachers taught me long ago that God is love. Genie, Tyler, Marion and I have felt God's love in abundance through your hugs, your tears, your wonderful letters and cards, your calls, beautiful flowers, delicious food, fantastic chocolate chip cookies, pictures and happy banners for my hospital room, but especially through your prayers. God has shown His love through you—and I love you for it! Now for a up-to-date report.*

> Physically - *I feel fantastic and look great for an*

old dude just six weeks over fifty. We have been hiking four to six miles every day for the last week. I could whip any hot-shot handball player if my doc would let me play. I have no loss of appetite, blood pressure is normal. In short, you would think that this guy is looking good.

Mentally - *From the moment I knew I had renal cell carcinoma, I went on the attack. There has been no depression, no anger, no fear, just desire to get the gears rolling. With the aid of the caring, fast-moving Greensboro medical community, we had the wheels turning in short order.*

Spiritually - *From the very beginning, I have had a sense of peace. I have prayed for strength and God has delivered that through family, our Pastor, close friends, my staff, and all of you who care. We feel very blessed.*

We've had a slight change of plans. The National Institutes of Health is no longer in the picture. We feel that Duke is the right place for us. I am scheduled to be at Duke next Tuesday, and we're hoping for some quick decisions on my treatment there. We will send you all a postcard to let you know firm plans and an address as soon as we get the word.

The Stones would like for you to help us in our challenge, and I am asking you to do the following things:

1. Please read the following verses from the Bible: Ps. 23:4, John 6:47, Prov. 8:17, Is. 55:12, Heb. 11:1, Jer. 30:17, Ps. 31:24, John 3:16, John 13:34,35, I John 4:19.

24

2. Please read some or all of the following books: Anatomy of An Illness, *and* Head First: The Biology of Hope *by Norman Cousins;* Love, Medicine,and Miracles *and* Peace, Love, and Healing *by Bernie Siegel, MD (also on tape);* Healing Yourself *By Martin Rossman, MD.*

3. Be thinking—when I get a hospital address, I would like for you to send me pictures—of you, your children, your grandchildren, your parents, your pets, your current girl or boy friends or friends; cards or letters telling me what you're doing, what's happening with your family, business, school, your career plans, who you think will be in the Final Four, funny stories. Think about making tapes reminding me of fun times we've had together, jokes, and the funniest thing that has ever happened to you (we hold everything in confidence). Draw pictures for my room. I want to smile and laugh a great deal!

4. Please send your leftover Girl Scout cookies. I understand my colleagues and the staff at the Duke Comprehensive Cancer Center have a ferocious appetite!!

5. Please call the weather station and leave us messages. We will have weather updates and I love to hear your voices.

6. Lastly, but most important, remember us in your prayers. You will certainly be in ours.
                                        Love, Bob

My reading list was not only designed to get people involved but it also (and it's a very important *also*) provided a common ground for later discussion, questions, etc. A reading list seemed to be one way of overcoming the shyness and fear of talking about a life-threatening illness. My team actually did read much of what was assigned. We all got a valuable update on the latest cancer treatments, we learned the lingo—white cells, C-cells, LAK—we learned to talk the game!

In my first letter, I invited more than 100 neighbors, friends, college pals, acquaintances, and work associates to become a part of my team. But numbers are not important. Like the Marine Corps you can do it with only a few good men. Suzanne Lewis did exactly that.

Suzanne was a Director with the Peace Corps in Gambia, West Africa when she was shipped post-haste back to the states with cancer and a harrowing medical prognosis. She was single, returning stateside for the first time in years, and many of her gang was over *there*, rather than here.

Undaunted, Suzanne did a fast study of the team concept. "Actually I thought it was a little *hokey* at first but I couldn't think of a better approach to let friends know I was sick and ask for their help." She drafted a letter, (many copies faxed between two continents) which was remarkable in its straight-forward, low-keyed approach. She asked for help—for prayers, for letters and cards, for encouragement. And Suzanne put together a team that did indeed see her through, all the way. She died a year later, but with the support and love and prayers of steadfast teammates. And it is my *hope* that Suzanne's adventure has only begun.

With that first letter in the mail, Genie and I loaded the car and headed straight up to the Blue Ridge Mountains. My father always said there was a lot of healing in those Carolina mountains. Walking four miles a day and eating at Genie's training table and breathing clean mountain air was just what Coach Genie prescribed to get ready for the surgery ahead, and all that lay beyond those mountains that we couldn't see from the valley.

FIVE

A Digression—
What They Knew and When

Even with the U.S. Postal Service on duty, bad news seldom travels a direct route. Bad news travels in wide, wheeling circles like a bird of prey, waiting, hovering, then swooping down from an untroubled, cloudless sky. How did the Buffaloes learn about the challenge they would all face together? The following vignettes tell us what they knew and when.

When Martha Stone Woods pulled into her drive that afternoon, her brother's shiny new four-wheel drive vehicle was parked in the turnaround. Her brother couldn't wait to show it off to his big sister when he got the monster two months ago. Bob and Martha were the only two in their family left now. Both parents rested in the family cemetery. Their sister Mary had died two years ago of lung cancer. That made for a special closeness between Bob and Martha.

Bob would stay over for supper, Martha decided, and watch the Hornets basketball game on television. Martha walked into the house and started mentally counting pork chops when she saw Genie was with Bob—and their son, Tyler, too. All of them were waiting for her in the vaulted living room overlooking pond and marsh.

But it was her brother's face that stopped Martha dead in her tracks.

"What?" she said.

"I've got cancer," Bob said.

"Where?"

"All over, everywhere—kidneys, liver, spleen, lungs. I'm eaten up with it." Bob looked at her, helpless and shaken, as if to say, "Don't you think our make-believe has gone on long enough?"

Martha had seen that look on Bob's face a hundred times. Bob, the good doctor, his toy stethoscope dangling over a sister prostrate with plague or polio or whatever. She remembered the time Mary had started to cry, caught up in her own make-believe. Seeing Mary's tears, Bob had yanked off his stethoscope to put an end to their game. Brother and sister clung to each other, locked in that moment of grief, afraid of that day when they would not be able to save each other. Martha saw that same look on her brother's face now.

Martha's bag of groceries slipped from her arms. Oranges caromed across the polished floor into broken broccoli and boxes of frozen dinners.

"I was playing handball at the "Y" last week," Bob began carefully. "I came up with blood in my urine—now that'll scare you pretty good. I called my urologist and he had me come in right away."

"Bob, they can do a lot with cancer now." Her brother was big and strong. It was impossible to believe that inside him so much was wrong. But Martha saw something in her brother's eyes that made her heart stop beating, a fragile but growing awareness that life might not be forever.

Jenny Stone Humphries was in the kitchen watching supper defrost in the microwave when her cousin Martha called. Martha relayed her terrible news, her voice tight and unsteady.

Later in helpless tears, Jenny agonized over how best to let another human being know you loved them, you were with them, that they *meant* something to you?

Reel after reel of grainy, herky-jerky home movies, made

through the years, bore witness to the bond she and her twin sister shared with their three cousins, Mary, Martha and Bob. Languid summer days, fragrant with figs from the bushes outside their screened porch in Charlotte, crisp Thanksgivings at their grandmother's home in Stoneville, where there were more cut-ups than the turkey; Christmases with dime store gifts and irrepressible high jinks.

This unholy alliance would see the cousins through the magic country of childhood to the gate that marked the rough terrain and flattened furrows of their adult years. There they had wished each other well and gone their separate ways. For a while. Then after the urgent demands of young families had abated, the cousins had found one another again. Family reunions, the weddings of their children, the leisure and hospitality of weekend homes. Mary's illness reconnected them so solidly that they could hardly remember *not* being together.

It was her cousin Mary's illness and death that had brought the families closer. Jenny and her husband were having a lazy Saturday morning brunch on the deck when the insistent ring of the telephone scattered the two bluejays waging war in the grape arbor.

"Jenny, this is Bob. Has Mary called you?"

Memory reformed five skinny kids piled into a red wagon, scratching chigger bites while grim mothers raked unruly hair smooth and smiled distractedly at the camera.

How could you ever lose touch with a wagon load of cousins like that, Jenny chastened herself. "I haven't heard from Mary. What's up?" Jenny asked.

"We've got one sick girl on our hands," Bob's voice had that competitive edge to it.

"What is it?"

"Her doctor's found a tumor."

Jenny had a instant memory snapshot of Mary with her hooded sad eyes, rueful grin, eloquent shrug from behind a veil of cigarette smoke.

"Breast?"

"No, it's in her lung and it's bad. She's being referred to

Emory. I'm driving down tonight."

Suddenly Bob Stone was as close as when the two cousins had been banished to the back steps for an infringement on adult rules.

"We're here and your bed is made."

Bob wheeled into the driveway at midnight. He refused the guest room and linen towels and French milled soap and climbed the stairs to a boy's room. Posters of Darth Vader and Star Wars, bookshelves crammed with models, an elaborate diorama spread out on a desk.

"My kind of room," Bob had laughed, stowing his hang-up bag in the closet.

The news from the hospital the next day was not good. "Terminal," Bob said over the pay phone, above the foreign noises of a hospital corridor. "They biopsied and it's lung cancer. No doubt about it."

"Does Mary know?" Jenny asked.

"She knows." There was more than those two words of pain in Bob's voice. "They gave her absolutely no hope."

Now it was Bob who had cancer. Jenny called Bob in Greensboro and got his answering service. The line to his office was constantly busy as friends and family tried to make that vital connection to a friend in deep trouble. More frustration the next day. Jenny gave up and wrote a letter. The letter didn't say all that was in her heart but she tried.

Jenny still carried the long-ago image of that sturdy little kid leaping out from the cover of a fig bush, dime-store six shooters blazing in the afternoon sun. BANG, BANG, YOU'RE DEAD!

Kathryn Reid had just come in from her ALTA tennis game in Dunwoody, Georgia when her sister Martha telephoned. "It's about Bob Stone," her sister began. Bob Stone! How long since she and John had heard from the Stones? *Ages.* Kathryn and her husband had explored Germany with Bob and Genie in the sixties. Both girls came from the same hometown of Chester, South Carolina; John and Bob, two GIs trying to do it all in one tour of duty—skiing, sight-seeing, trading at the PX. The two couples had kept up haphazardly through the years. How could you lose touch with friends like that, Kathryn chided herself.

Kathryn was suddenly aware of the tension in her sister's voice. "Bob has cancer. I heard it from a friend in Charlotte."

Unable to reach Bob, Kathryn had to make do with with a message left on Bob's answering machine. Days later she received Bob's first letter. "He wants us to be on his team," she said handing her husband Bob's letter. And for the second time in their lives she and John were going to war with the Stones. And she was betting there were lots more out there who would be joining them.

SIX

Rocky Start to a Long Season

I took possession of my hospital bed on the seventh floor of the cancer wing at the Duke University Medical Center; the Jordan Ward it is called. I told myself that the best thing I had going for me was that I was not the complete package; throw in Genie and Marion and Tyler and *still* you didn't have the complete package. I had a team. That's what I kept telling myself. I had an edge in my battle against cancer.

I had sent out a hundred letters in that first draft of friends, family, fellow travelers and odd balls. I had to believe they were out there. Otherwise I would have been a bonafide, *pro quid*, certifiable nut. And I had enough to contend with already without that.

I was feeling shaky with my surgery only a couple of days away. It would have been so easy to give myself over to the anxiety and apprehension of what lay ahead. And one of the most potent psychological weapons against any threat is the power of *many*. Isolation, loneliness, and depression, fear dissipate when it is spread out among the *many*. I had already sensed that when I felt the support of friends that afternoon in my kitchen, grazing among a plenty of casseroles and good wishes. Now I was waiting to see how many friends, associates, former Davidson classmates, fellow committee persons, church members would answer my call.

Even under the best of circumstances, the whole process of

hospitalization was somewhat dehumanizing. I gave the Duke staff an A plus. They go all out to make you feel like a Me, not a Thing. Sure these people are trained to handle their patients efficiently, but no training could teach them to care like they do. The staff on the seventh floor were the pick of the litter.

Hospitals are not designed to be overwhelming. It just happens. There are arrows directing you along miles of corridors, to other wings, into other buildings. You frantically decode unfamiliar signage. Hospitals, which are meant to be a tower of help and healing, often become a tower of Babel. At least here at the Duke Cancer Center they send along a guide to bring you through the wilderness, a volunteer with the cancer support group. That's how we met Nancy Emerson. She had more to offer than a sunny smile. She'd been there. She knew first-hand about cancer. And she had won.

From high atop the Jordan Ward, I looked glumly at Genie. "It's a nice place to visit but I wouldn't want to live here."

Genie would have none of that kind of talk. This was a gal who left the considerable comforts of home for the challenge of an Outward Bound experience. This was the gal who, over the years, took seven foster infants into our home to love. This was the woman who opened her home and her heart to a homesick black preacher from Haiti while he was recovering from surgery. Genie Stone was open to adventure—even here on this floor of seriously sick folks. Genie likes falling off mountains. You might call it rappelling—I call it falling!

Genie and Marion had taken a room nearby so they could walk to the hospital and share the duty watch. I looked down from my window and saw Marion, her knapsack of books and healthy snacks slung over her shoulder, dodging traffic in the street below. Silky haired, tall, and serene, her appearance was one of fragileness but her stamina was the stuff that got the wagons across the mountains and westward.

Always my quiet enigmatic child, Marion brought into my hospital room a feeling of peace and hope that was fierce. She brought a breath of freshness when she came on the floor, dropping in on other patients, sharing the lore of those who have

33

learned how to wait...and wait.

"It's going to be important how we handle this," she had said that day she got off the plane that brought her home from Montana. "Grieving isn't all bad," she said, quietly acknowledging that grief is a necessary part of coming to grips with cancer. This tall, economy-worded young woman had laid it out on the table. This is serious. Let's not pretend. I know so many people—husbands and wives, kids and parents—who just can't bring themselves to talk about the issue. They fall silent, they talk banalities. But Marion brought the subject of cancer out in the open. I learned something from her. We were all in this thing together and it was better to talk than play Let's Pretend. Quiet Marion had managed to jack up communication skills between father and daughter a couple of proud notches.

Genie paid no attention to my melancholy appraisal of our new home away from home. She had a surprise. Genie briskly unfurled a banner for the bare wall. Smile faces and a logo which read: Have A Good Day!!! The computer banner was an explosion of primary colors—actually an explosion of Hassenfelts—five lively girls, ages five to sixteen who lived next door to us.

So my team from Nowhere was answering my first call for support. In the days ahead, my generic hospital room was transformed into a joint that rocked with good will and caring!

In my first letter I'd asked for some very specific things—prayers, photographs, recycled jokes. And my team was responding!

A charter team member, Peggy Shuford, in Hickory, sent a huge wall map, PEOPLE, PLACES, & PRAYERS. Red flags marked the homes of team members across the country. Snapshots, gag shots, and long shots were what the team was dealing from the Jordan Ward of the Duke Comprehensive Cancer Center.

Good communications are a must in getting a team off and running. Where you are exactly—hospital, West Africa, or Oz—and what is happening *now* is Need To Know Information and makes team members feel a vital part of the whole. Communications make the team! But building good communications takes enormous effort. "There were times," Genie will tell you, her brown eyes reflecting the pain of rough days, "when it all just seemed too much--keeping up with the letters, the telephone calls—but when you saw how much they meant, you managed to get it done somehow. Teams don't just happen!" Genie smiles wistfully.

Genie is right. Teams don't just *happen.* Our team was going to need a good communications network to relay important information. I realized I would have to look ahead to what was coming up so I could fire off my *bon mots* before surgery or scheduled treatment. That way I could feel the muscle of all that good will and support behind me on those days when life wasn't going according to Roberts Rules of Order. And what about my family? They could certainly use a little TLC to keep them going.

Just before the surgery to remove my cancerous kidney, I sent out a second letter to the team, giving our mailing addresses and publicizing our opening round of competition against my worthy opponent.

Dear Family and Friends,
LET THE GAMES BEGIN!
Q. When do the games begin?
A. March 22, 1990
Q. Where are the Opening ceremonies being held?
A. Duke University Cancer Center.
Q. What is the first event?
A. Radical nephrectomy of a wonderful, but tired left kidney.
Q. What is the time of the event?
A. Friday morning, March 23.
Q. Where will the team reside?
A. Our address is:
Q. From a long-time Charlotte/Davidson friend—
Will there be writs or review on the Bible verses or books recommended?

35

A. Your work is pledged.
Q. What kind of jokes shall I send in? Are one-liners okay?
A. Sure. It's better to have loved a short girl than never love a tall.
Q. From a homely-looking high school buddy—will my baby picture do?
A. Absolutely—I prefer it!
Q. How long will the first event last?
A. The team will be at Duke until March 30.
Q. What is the next venue?
A. Four to six weeks training at the beach and in the mountains.
Q. What next?
A. Back to Duke for the main event. Friendly competition with the protocol.
Q. How long will it last?
A. Two weeks.
Q. What are side effects?
A. I'll look like the Pillsbury Dough Boy or the Michelin Tire Man for awhile, but I understand the wide look is coming back in.
Q. How do we get an update?
A. Call the weather station.
Q. Do Bob, Genie, Tyler and Marion love you?
A. ABSOLUTELY--and we appreciate your continued support!

Love, Bob

With each letter, I was trying to build a base of shared humor and empathy. Cancer itself cannot be shared with everyone (thank God!) but humor and caring can be. You learn to sympathize, empathize, synthesize.

Even unorthodox teams like the one I was putting together get bonded in these three ways.

You *sympathize*. Poor guy, bad things really do happen to good people. Try this honest I-fell-down-and-hurt-my-knee approach at any good playground and see what you get. A crowd of sympathizers, that's what!

Then you *empathize*. I-know how-I'd feel-if-this-were happening-to-me-and-here's-what-I'd-do! Empathy does not require high-tech skills or an impressive vitae. Anyone can do it. It's called Walk A Mile In My Shoes. Even if the one you are sympathizing and empathizing with is ensnared in an unimaginable situation, you can still break down the unimaginable into imaginable pieces. Can't imagine AIDS? Can you imagine not feeling like cooking dinner tonight or, even worse, not eating dinner tonight? You get the idea.

The endgame is when we *synthesize* all this deepening compassion and insight out into our larger world—a world out there that's bigger than just you and me. Open the locks and see where the force of caring thrusts you. You may find yourself approaching universal concerns with a fresh and healing vision of what you can do to help.

During the time I was settling into the routine of the Jordan Ward I was talking *team* to everyone who dropped by and was impacted by our posters, cards and banners. My team was an all-purpose conversation starter to personalize the impersonal, to keep anxiety and apprehension on a tight leash.

I talked *team* non-stop to these caregivers. If they could care about me, I reasoned, then I could care about them enough to make contact with the human being underneath that starched white uniform, a person who was pretty much like me right down to our immune system and renal cells!

And that's exactly what I tried to do with every doctor, intern, nurse, and aide who came into my room. I asked about their work, their kids, their family, their significant other, what teams they liked, how they managed their cholesterol in the face of terminal chocolate chip cookies. In turn, I opened up my own life, letting others get a real good gander at this fellow, who, from the brevity of his hospital gown, looked like he'd been seriously short-sheeted!

WHERE THE BUFFALOES ROAM

I found that Bernie Siegel and Norman Cousins were right. Laughter was my best medicine. Laughter put the staff at ease, it put my visitors at ease, and, last but not least, it took my mind off the upcoming surgery, umpteen lab tests, much drawing of blood and vital fluids.

Somewhere in this process of talking *team*, I discovered nurses, aides, eager interns, sleep-deprived residents, and the big docs themselves were vying to be on my team. What better way for them to deal with the less than optimum conditions they faced every day? If you can't beat this guy and his team of banner artists and map makers, why not join them? And that is exactly what they did.

It was one of the nurses on our team, who let it drop that my surgeon, Dr. Philip Walther, was a chocolate freak. That started the fun. Since he was the fellow doing the carving, it made sense for me to sweeten my position in any way I could. I sent Marion scurrying for two boxes of deluxe, imported chocolates—the kind you *hope* for when no one's looking. One box went to the floor nurses to bribe them to join me in a little D-Day madness. The deal was sweet: as soon as I was tranquilized and on my way down to surgery, a nurse was to position the box of chocolates under my surgical sheet.

I wasn't actually "there" when Dr. Walther uncovered his "glory hole" but I was told his grin said it all. The doc removed one left kidney, assorted tumors and two hazelnut clusters in record time. All in a morning's work!

Pro football players are always complaining about the "big cut." My big cut was about eighteen inches long, running across mid field. Assorted tubes, drains and surgical staples littered the playing field. A radical nephrectomy should head everyone's Must Miss list.

I used my newly-learned skill of visualization to help me manage the pain following surgery. I imagined calm, restful places. I saw myself strong and healthy, doing things I'd done when I was in peak condition—playing handball. (I must be a demon for punishment. You would think I'd never want to see one of those hard rubber balls again.)

I tried to focus on wonderful times with my family, my friends. I imagined my team lining up behind me—and what do you know—I looked up and there they were!

My Big Three, Vic, Larry and David, were on hand that first day the nurse got me up after my surgery. Even now I wince at the memory. I had this drainage tube which was unbelievably painful, worse than the incision. The guys came trooping in, wanting so badly to help me. I mean they were a *wall* of male support you could lean on. And I did. Larry saw my pain was running off the Richter scale. "We'll pray for you Bob." he said.

"No," I gasped, "let me pray. I'll go first." I was all hunkered over in a chair, trying to draw a breath without breathing. "Jesus wept." I panted, reciting the shortest Bible verse in the Bible, and one which pretty well described my own state. The guys broke up. What a boost that gave me, seeing that all of us could still laugh—no, make that *some* of us could still laugh.

The "Jesus wept" story was told and passed around until it became a part of the team lore. Like any other team, our team was beginning to share stories, jokes, even cartoons. We were developing a persona!

SEVEN

Prize Offer

During the course of my illness I had long hours to explore creative approaches to handling big problems. Visualization, meditation, prayer are all means of tapping into the creative powers we have within ourselves. It has been surprising how my wife and I have come to look at these spiritual resources. Before my illness I think it would be fair to say that Genie was more open than myself to innovative, creative ways of living her life. She is a creative person. She dances, paints professionally, can shape and throw a clay pot with the best of them. Genie can do anything with her hands. She was very interested in many alternative spiritual resources. As for me, with seven generations of tall, big-boned Calvinists behind me, including a Dad who was a minister, I was predictably orthodox in my backup systems.

Prayer, visualization, and meditation all have the ability to calm the mind, soothe and enlarge our sense of well-being. I am working hard for my proficiency badge in all three. Case studies exploring the phenomenon of self-healing indicate that the more open and curious a person is, the better his chance of beating overwhelming odds; he doesn't close his mind to any reasonable possibility. My own resource manual is the Bible and it validates this very kind of openness when it instructs us that we must become as children—to me that means wide-eyed, innocent and excited about life—a walking exclamation point!

But as I have moved deeper into this challenge of pain, discouragement, and even death, I found myself becoming less and less orthodox while Genie was becoming more so. Now I listen with courteous interest when the talk turns to crystals, positive imaging, alternative medicine. But I have something even better to offer. Corinthians tells us the greatest gift we have is love; I'd like to add another. Prayer. Both Genie and I agree.

During exhausting and often painful treatment, prayer was a solid powerful force I tapped into again and again. Good prayer is like drafting behind Richard Petty on a good day at the Charlotte Motor Speedway. You can feel its thrust, lock into its power, glide into a slot where things become a little more possible.

I would be the first to agree that prayer doesn't always offer the quick fix or the fast save. There are times when the pain does not go away, ominous shadows do not vanish, hours and hours of waiting are still interminable. But what both Genie and I have discovered is that with good honest prayer and with nothing else, comes an abiding sense that you have not been abandoned. Whether you are lying in ICU, locked into destructive habits, or enmeshed in the deep weeds of a major problem, prayer may not be a cure-all but it does give a peace that nothing else can give. And there is no greater comfort than the feeling that you have not been abandoned and left alone.

When friends who have listened and laughed with me over the years gathered around and said "let's pray," they were offering me a power as solid as the front line of the Steelers. Not a single one of us could lay claim to a Nobel prize or a McArthur grant for genius, but our simple, honest prayers were a force to be reckoned with. In her openness to other possibilities, Genie found that earnest prayer was a life line she could depend on.

I found that I was not the only one reaping support from my team. Genie and the kids were beneficiaries, as well. They needed the steadfast support and strength of a team as much or more than I did.

This was especially true for my son Tyler. Unlike Marion who was just out of college, Tyler was already launched on his career path. His time and his energy were already spoken for. He provided stalwart help and support to the family on the weekends but where was his support during the time he was not with us? He discovered his friends wanted to be a part of my team for that very reason––to support him during his own crisis. What a wonderful and valuable thing for young men to learn together–– friending.

A phone call, a card or letter, a message left on the weather station for Genie or one of the kids, a drop-in visitor with a sack of deli sandwiches let them know they were being supported in their big challenge too. That's what a "team" is all about. Every guy on the team gets the same consideration, the same respect for his needs as the quarterback.

Every team needs a tangible prize or goal to set their sights on—a Super Bowl ring, a weenie roast after the big game, a weekend at the beach, a yearly blowout at the local pub. Competitions, prizes, contests can light a spark that ignites a team-sized conflagration. My cousin Jenny lit a fire under me when she came up with a prize offer that produced a stampede of Buffaloes chasing a red bike!

Jenny's prize offer arrived in a large envelope emblazoned with the jargon of sweepstakes mania: BOB STONE YOU ARE DEFINITELY A WINNER! PLEASE CLAIM YOUR PRIZE! PRIZE WINNING NUMBER ENCLOSED! Jenny made me an offer I couldn't refuse.

Wednesday, March 21, 1990

Dear Bob,

After your call I realized that we are really messing up big time. We've let you go up against the Duke Medical juggernaut without selecting our marching song, the music we will be known by. Even little David was accompanied by a lyre. Bob, we've got to have an anthem which will identify our Movement. All the good movements have them. "We Shall Overcome" comes readily to mind but it's been done to death. I believe you will agree that our anthem should sound the ringing Calvinist tones of our faith. What we want is a song that is Presbyterian but also just a little raunchy. I offer my nomination, Keith Whitley's It Ain't Nothing. *You guys who belong to the Pickup and RV crowd may be all over this one but just in case a tape is enclosed. I think it sort of fits a Bob Stone—laid back, an easy rhythm which is of crucial importance in your present situation, if I read you.*

In my earlier letter we talked about winning and prizes. But details were omitted. You have convinced me that you are serious about winning so let's go for the gold. There is really only one prize worth winning.

IT'S A SCHWINN, BOB!
This bike is being offered through a special arrangement with the Schwinn Company, official outfitters of Stone Expeditions for half a century.

The bike is fully loaded and customized to your exact specifications. It is turbo-charged. The brakes have been stripped from this particular model so that upon reaching optimum racing speed there is, quite literally, no stopping you.

It comes with fringed driving gloves and white sidewall sneakers with steel toes (remember no brakes).

Custom trim kit includes two squirrel tails for the handlebars. Pony skin saddle seat for that touch of pure luxury. Aerial for your flag (It goes whoosh, whoosh!). Included as standard equipment are two clothespins and a pack of Bicycle playing cards which also make snazzy wheel covers. Mud flaps with 2 glo-lite glass studs for inclement weather complete the package.

Other lesser prizes: Sylvester Stallone's boxing trunks, a lifetime subscription to GRIT, the bestseller, The Six Week Cholesterol Cure *(the remedy is severe, as you already know first hand), a heavy duty truss (for when things start slipping). We even offer a splendid consolation prize: Eternal Glory (awarded with two (2) Oak Leaf Clusters).*

But Bob the prize you want is the bike. It's red.

Love, Jenny

Naturally a prize as terrific as the red bike didn't just happen. You guessed it, there's a story here. Jenny confesses all. "Bob responded with such spirit to Field Marshall Foch's feisty communication that I rummaged through my mind for another incentive. What we needed was a prize, it had to be symbolic—resonating with the high spirits of better days—and most of all the prize had to be real enough to trip an adrenalin surge that would give Bob the big push over that first big hurdle."

Jenny went puddle-jumping back through our childhood. She remembered that prince of commerce who knocked on the front door with a big grin every Saturday morning to ante up. She remembered the news carrier who hustled enough to win his share of contests put on by the *Charlotte Observer*. I was that gofer. I'd won ball gloves, footballs, movie passes. Just mention the word *prize* and my blood would come up to simmer.

An undamaged cluster of memories filed deep in her cerebellum provided Jenny with what she was looking for. Jenny remembered the summer of the Texas evangelist and his wonderful prize.

The preacher had left Texas heavenbent on laying waste to sin and the devil's work with his Kids Campaign. Get 'em while they're young, before the devil has his way with them. He had set himself up on the steps of Central High School in Charlotte. The turnout had been disappointing. The city was locked in the irons of summer heat and sin. Esther Williams and Fernando Lamas were cavorting at the local drive-in, both of them in swimsuits like *skin!* The preacher was down to riding the rims in this series of revival meetings. Even the humidity was against him. And at 25 cents a gallon for gasoline, this trip doing the Lord's work was proving to be anything but economical. The evangelist needed some way to drum up business.

A prize! Sure! He'd promote an extra special night and the youth who brought the most folks to his kid campaign would win a super prize...something on the order of a...a bike! Gosh yes, what red-blooded, All-American kid wouldn't want to win a bicycle!

The preacher went shopping. "I'm sure this red Schwinn is just what you have in mind," the salesman said, running his hand over the gleaming chrome and brilliant red paint. The preacher studied his shoes. The Lord hadn't seen fit to give him enough financial resources for this top-of-the-line model. "Maybe something a little less expensive," the evangelist hedged. "But you've got the right idea! I sure would like it to be red."

The salesman executed a quick reverse and rolled out a no-name bike to fit the preacher's limited resources. This bike was so red it didn't need a name!

Of course, I wanted it. This bike. Because it was free, because it was brand new, because it was fire-engine red. I could almost hear the clatter of playing cards clothespinned to the wheel. I could see a snazzy pair of raccoon tails flying from the handlebars.

"I can get you the numbers," my dad volunteered. "I'm working in the projects in south Charlotte this week and there's plenty of souls waiting to be claimed for the Lord, if you can figure out how to get them across town."

I tore up the stairs to my bedroom and dug my savings bank out of a drawer. I calculated I had enough dimes to buy tokens for two bus loads of kids. But how could I keep them happy enough to make sure I could deliver them all the way? A box of Tootsie Pops took care of that. "Get right on board," I shouted, handing each kid a sucker and a big grin. The kids campaign shifted into turbo-glide. The kids were ecstatic—a free bus ride with the windows wide open on a muggy night and dessert included!

That night everyone won big. The Texas evangelist won. The Lord won. One hundred and fifty kids won. And I won, hands down. I even forgave the red bike for not being a Schwinn.

So now our team had something to go after, a red bike to rally around. With Jenny's prize offer on the table, this former news carrier really got pedaling. Bob Stone caught the fever. This team had something going—the sizzle of that shiny red Schwinn that every kid had wanted in the year B.C. (Before Chevys).

I saw the prize and the competition to win it as a metaphor for my fight against cancer. Could I win the red bike? Could I beat cancer? It clicked in my mind. Besides, competition for a red bike had more glitz than a dull readout on my white cell count.

I could see the team rallying behind me for the big win. Yes, we had a TEAM! We had a prize the—gosh, my team didn't have an official name! I'd been so busy laying the groundwork for the new team, I'd forgotten about a name.

Deciding on the name *Buffaloes* for our team was a natural. I have to come clean and confess that my nickname in college was Buffalo Bob. In my student days, I sold ads in the Davidson football programs, hawked tickets to Homecoming, detailed the splendors of a senior class ring—you name it—just a preacher's boy trying to make his date money. Some of my classmates claimed I was a genetic throwback to those frontier traders who brokered in hides, wampum, tobacco, and beads, so they started calling me Buffalo Bob. But from a broader perspective, you couldn't help but respect a breed of animal still hanging in there after a couple of hundred years. Tough old Buffaloes were what we were!

In the days that followed my surgery, I thought often about those patient critters who had perversely outlasted their own extinction. They had made it. So could I. As soon as I was operative following my surgery, I wasted no time in giving chase to the red bike and asking my teammates to join me.

April 5, 1990

Dear Family and Friends,

There were six bright, pretty, very verbal and extremely humorous granddaughters in the Stone Family when I arrived in 1940. My two sisters and four cousins welcomed me with loving opened arms, because I brought to their creative world of play the one missing ingredient—a male. The summertimes we spent together were full of fun and adventure. I would do anything they wanted me to do with a smile, because the girls convinced me that's what the role of a little brother/cousin should be. I worked a lot. I can remember my mother playing a jazzed-up wedding march on the piano, as I was the preacher, the groom, and ring bearer in one of our many gala weddings! In short, these young ladies were and still are world-class motivators. Jenny's done it again, folks. I WANT THAT RED BIKE!

On March 16, I wrote to you asking to help the Stones with our challenge and listed some things to do. Today I'm asking you to join the team that now has an organizational structure. Before giving you the specifics let me tell you how the Opening Ceremonies turned out.

The Duke University Medical Staff showed up in its finest regalia and performed a world-class radical nephrectomy in record time (3 1/2 hours, I am told). The nursing staff was the best! Their professional ability along with a loving, caring manner helped me and my family get through some rough waters. The atmosphere at Duke is perfect for healing.

My room did not look like a hospital room at all except for some fellow in the bed hooked up to a lot of hoses. Your drawings, cards, flowers, banners, and especially the photographs made my room the brightest in all of Duke Hospital. Some friends from Hickory sent a 3'x4' map of the USA entitled "Stone Camp—People, Places, & Prayers." We put flags where all you folks live. My room was a happy place to visit and I thank you for it!

Now for the specific data on OUR TEAM.

The General Manager and Team Physician—The Lord God

As General Manager, He has been impressed with our showing in the first event. As the Team Physician, His fee is small, but His work is priceless.

Head Coach—Genie Stone

Assistant Head Coaches—Tyler and Marion Stone

Team Name—The Buffaloes

Prize Offer

Tough ole dudes with a will to live, as evidenced by their remarkable comeback over the last 100 years.

Genie, Tyler, Marion and I thank you for your continued loving support.

Love, Bob
I Corinthians 13:13

That letter brought an immediate visible response from John Sebrell in Virginia. He fired off a bundle of five hundred bumper stickers proclaiming the Buffaloes UNDEFEATABLE CHAMPS.

So now this team was more than an idea. We were a reality, an entity. The Buffaloes were a real team. We had a name. We had a prize worth going after.

EIGHT

Playing With the Big Boys

We reached a quick consensus on the naming of our team. Jean Winje, an old friend, voiced immediate approval:

Bob,

I agree on the team name: The Buffaloes. So I talked with the U.S. Postal Service and they agreed to print up a billion of these cards—just to honor the team!!!

Jeannie's note was written on the newly-issued "America the Beautiful" postal card with the buffalo stamp!

The Buffaloes had been officially named, stars marking their homes on our official team map, their names emblazoned on bumper stickers. The team was ready to get down and play some ball with the big boys at the Duke Comprehensive Cancer Center. They had proved that they could turn a dreary hospital room into an oasis of hope and humor, but that was just a warm-up.

April 23, 1990

Dear Team,

LET THE GAMES CONTINUE!

Q. When do they begin?
A. As you read this, our team, the Buffaloes, is on the offensive and attacking the cancer with the best gameplan known for kidney cancer: Interleukin-2 plus LAK cells.
Q. What is the current score?
A. The Buffaloes - 97 Cancer - 3
The surgery on March 23rd removed 97% of the cancer which was located in the left kidney and several lymph nodes. We need to work on the remaining 3% so that the Final Score will be: The Buffaloes - 100 Cancer - 0.
Q. How do we win?
A. In short, a TEAM effort
   1. Faith in God
   2. Faith in our medical team and IL-2
   3. Positive attitudes
   4. Prayer
Q. How can we learn more about IL-2?
A. The May issue of Ladies Home Journal *has an article, "Lee Remick's Quiet Fight," which describes exactly what IL-2 is and the recovery process. Ms. Remick, like the Stones, is fortunate to have had strong support from family and friends. It is a good article.*
Q. Isn't the plural of Buffalo Bison?
A. Yes. But Go-o-o-o Buffaloes sounds better than Go-o-o-Bison!
Q. Have the Stones been smiling and laughing?
A. Absolutely! Your cards, letters, photos, tapes, videos, cartoons of The Far Side, Calvin and Hobbes, Cathy, numerous jokes, You're a Redneck If, Anguished English, *and other books have kept us laughing. I have them all with me now and will need them over the next two weeks!*
Q. Did Craig Shergold break the Guinness Book of World Records?

A. Yes. With the help of most of you team members, Craig shattered the old record of 1,265,000 with over 5,000,000 cards, as of April 20. The Children's Wish Foundation expects that he will eventually receive over seven million cards. Thanks for helping.

Q. Should we look over our reading list again?

A. Yes. Reading the scripture verses again and again has helped me. Also, Head First, the Biology of Hope *by Norman Cousins is excellent, and you will be glad you read it.*

Q. Are you charging to see the scar?

A. Yes. $1.00 to the public—FREE to Team Members!

Q. What is my wish?

A. My wish is that I could thank each one of you personally for what you have meant to me, Genie, Tyler, and Marion over the last two months. God has shown us His love through each of you—It has been a wonderful experience. It is my hope that in the future we may be able to return God's love to you, a loved one, or a friend, if a life-threatening disease is experienced. We have learned that you cannot deny the diagnosis, but with faith in God, medical technology and the will to live, you can defy the outcome.

Q. Where does the Red Mountain Bike come in?

A. When I win the bike, you can ride it anytime. It's a fine bike!

Love, Bob
Romans 8:37-39

You can tell from my letter that our team was really getting comfortable with one another and gaining a sense of what we were doing here—facing crisis situations together. The team concept was working. So many of my own doubts and questions were being answered in such positive ways. Would anyone answer my call to join a team to help one guy face the biggest challenge of his life, I had wondered. Who really had time in their frenetic daily life to take on a guy and his family who was asking for a lot more than a place on your Christmas card list or a gift for the alumni building fund. With child rearing, graduations, weddings, school and career decisions, business demands, the torque of our individual lives can be crushing.

But we were all learning a lot. I discovered that people want to be connected, want to live and work and love something outside of themselves. This need in our human condition was translating itself into a team that only needed to be told where and when. You could count on them to be there.

There was much talk about "the protocol" at Duke. What exactly was *medical protocol,* the team wanted to know after I'd mentioned it in one of my letters. The Buffaloes knew about team doctors, trainers—but what was this medical protocol? One Buffalo came up with the answer. A doctor must formally ask my permission before killing me. That was close.

Dr. Philip Walther, my doctor at Duke, understood the protocol. He did ask my permission. "This IL-2 Plus LAK Cells is the most advanced weapon we've got against renal cell carcinoma," Dr. Walther told me. "It's also very toxic to the body. It's going to be like the worst case of the flu you've ever had."

I didn't know it then, but that was the good news. I was still weak from my nephrectomy but anxious to begin treatment so those C Cells would have more to contend with than a guy with a team of oddballs, one gallant kidney and a Bible.

I wanted my immune system to unleash its Star Wars capability. I was getting good at visualization. I closed my eyes and beamed up an opening battle. Laser tracers streaked across the screen of my mind, homing in on a cluster of cancer cells; I saw clouds of healing white smoke, cancer cells dropping like dead flies. This was war straight out of the book of Revelations where doom was written across the heavens in fiery tongues of flame while white-robed armies massed for all-out war. My field general was Pacman, state-of-the art warrior for state-of-the-art treatment.

I believed that visualization and positive imaging could be a powerful adjunct to the IL-2 treatment. During the time I was the sickest, I tried to focus on the IV that was dripping in huge doses of sickness and torment and think to myself, "This is good stuff! It's making me sick but go right ahead and shoot it to me because it's killing those cancer cells."

Using visualization techniques as a tool to focus the power of the mind to master your own personal challenges is one all of us might explore. Psychoneuroimmunology (remember that word!) is dependent on this kind of positive imaging. I asked my whole team to give it a try. Think of one person focusing on one thing, then multiply that by the number of your teammates all focusing together on the problem. Mind-boggling mind power! It makes harnessing the sun seem like child's play.

I found this concept of positive imaging and visualization tremendously exciting, not a lot of hocus-pocus. Studies suggest that those with open, inquiring minds are most successful in defeating illness. And with my prognosis, an open inquiring mind was about the only thing I had going for me. It seemed to me that visualization was not a new world but simply a new creative way of looking at my world. I was still the same fellow under that warm shower, whacking the devil out of that handball, but visualization did offer a positive and fresh way of relating to the world I lived in. And who knows, maybe it really was a powerful weapon and cancer-killer extraordinaire.

And I found I really needed all the extra darts I could lay hands on in this game they called IL-2. The first week of IL-2 went great. But when they began to feed those souped-up cancer-killer cells back into my body all hell broke loose. I was sick, feverish, aching, itching, fighting the afflictions of Job—and losing, it seemed to me. I was dimly aware of a crowd of doctors gathered around my aching body as my medical status was downgraded from "tolerable" to "iffy". I barely remember that fast fade to black.

I was very weak when they wheeled me into ICU with a blood pressure of 50/30 and kidney failure. All I could think of was the Buffaloes out there pulling for me, investing so much effort in both me and my family. I knew my team wasn't going to give up on me, so in a reverse backlash of team pride I had no choice but to hang in there for my team. "Suck it up, you wimp!" I told myself. "You can't let the team down."

For all of you out there thinking about putting your own challenge team together you should be aware of this danger: You've got your team for your challenge. You brought them together. They are your team. You feel a swell of pride when you think of them. They are there for you. But don't be surprised one day when the team you brought together turns the table. Suddenly you find they are not your team, you are *their* team. They call the plays, tell you what to do, critique your performance, exert a tremendous power over your conscious and unconscious mind. That's what I learned while hallucinating on the brink of the great unknown in ICU.

I was all by myself in the stands after a big football game. The crowds had gone, the playing field was deserted. There was just me in a great huge stadium with one stupendous mess of trashed pizza boxes, mustard-stained paper napkins, crushed drink cups. The job clearly called for a waste management team the size of the US Marine Corps. "Hey," I was pleading into this vast emptiness, "You can't leave me here with this mess! Give me a hand here, fellows!" But no help was offered. I labored away at this thankless grunt work barely making a dint in the pile of refuse. On and on I worked—stacking, sweeping, picking up. I was overwhelmed with a crushing realization that my team was depending on me to get this mess cleaned up. I couldn't walk away from my responsibility. I couldn't let them down, so on and on I sweated and toiled, hour after hour, working my heart out for the team.

It was much later that I was able to put the pieces of that nightmare together and understand what it meant. I couldn't let my team down. They weren't mine, I was theirs. I had no choice but to dig in. I couldn't leave them. They had invested too much time and effort for me to run off and leave them to live the rest of their lives happily ever after. I was discovering for myself the heartbreak of being a part of a team. All for one and one for all.

What kind of support can a team offer someone flat on his back in a hospital room with no view? To a large extent that depends on the physical condition of the one needing your support. In my own case I was in ICU during each of my three IL- 2 treatments. Most of that time during the treatment my condition was so precarious that visitors and drop-ins were not only discouraged but prohibited. And Genie and my family were so exhausted that what they needed most was to be left alone to rest and recoup for the next day.

My IL-2 Plus LAK treatments became a brutal marathon relay. Genie would tough it out as long as she could, then Marion would take over, then Tyler on the weekend, my sister Martha as needed. It was a grueling test of endurance and love because it involved so much hands-on care and physical handling. I was sick in every way that a human being can be sick—fever, nausea, diarrhea, hives. Our son Tyler caught his share of all this dross when he took over on the weekends. It was tough duty for a young man who once barfed when he spied mold in a left-over carton of whipped topping. I was worse than mold!

Once I awakened and found myself out of ICU and back in my own room. Tyler was sprawled in a chair, caved-in with fatigue. With a shock I realized my boy had become a man. What a lonely rite-of-passage this son had made—unheralded, fraught with uncertainty, through solitary hours of darkness and with first light of dawn as he drove back to Charlotte after those weekends—and through it all, with a grin and optimism that was his banner into the battle, a strength we all could depend on. I stirred and Tyler was at my bedside. "Need something, Dad?"

I couldn't think of a thing.

56

Support continued to pour in from the most astonishing and random channels.

Years ago, at a party, a friend who was an orthopedic surgeon had been discussing the abysmal quality of medical care in underdeveloped countries. "As a matter of fact," he told me, "I'm bringing over this preacher from Haiti." He went on to explain how a botched-up job on a broken leg had made the man into a cripple. "I'm flying him over for the operation he needs," the orthopedist confided. "Now I've got to find him a place to stay for a couple of weeks."

Genie dropped her stuffed pea pod. My wife is a sucker for a well executed Statue of Liberty play. Bring me your tired, your poor, your weary...somewhere in this world there are seven kids Genie took into our home, to give them all the love they needed.

"We'll take your preacher in," Genie volunteered. "We'd love to have him wouldn't we, Bob?"

We would and we did. Now this same minister in Haiti was writing to tell us that the members of his little church were praying for me around the clock.

I remember one particularly rough time during my second round of IL-2. I was back in ICU. I bobbed up out of drugged oblivion with something cold and hard pressed against my ear. Go ahead and pull the trigger, I thought weakly. But it was only a telephone receiver the ICU nurse was pressing against my ear. "Don't talk. Just listen," my nurse cautioned.

"Bob, this is Martha." There was no mistaking my sister's voice. She seemed very put-out with her brother. "Bob, they say you're not doing too good. Bob you just can't die and leave me alone. I've just had all I can take. First Mary, now you. Don't you go and die on me too, Bob Stone. Promise me. Bob, you absolutely *cannot* die on me, you hear? Just say yes, Bob."

"Yes," I barely croaked.

"That's good, Honey. Now you try to get some rest. I'm going to drive down to spell Genie as soon as school is out this afternoon. You keep thinking LIVE!"

I didn't dare *not* live. My sister is a very determined individual. I had seen just how determined years before, when our father suffered a massive stroke. Robbed of his speech, unable to communicate, my sister was the one who understood the heart of a man who had spent his life in the pulpit.

We were both at Dad's bedside that Sunday morning when he suddenly became restless and agitated. He fought to speak, a hopeless stream of gibberish coming from his lips. Again and again he tried to get her to understand. "Daddy, are you trying to preach?" my sister asked, operating strictly on intuition. She turned to me. "It's Sunday, Bob, Daddy wants to be in church."

Dad made a strangulated sound that Martha took as agreement. Then my sister performed an amazing act of pure love. She began to lead us through the simple Presbyterian church service my father knew like a North Carolina road map. "I'll sing," she announced, after my father came to a stopping place in his garbled sermon. Martha began to sing a familiar hymn in that quiet hospital room. Dad visibly relaxed. But after the hymn, he became agitated again. "Now for this morning's scripture lesson." Martha announced quickly, "Read a passage from the Bible, Bob." And so it went right on to the taking of the offering. My sister sang an offertory solo acappello. Step by step, we went through the order of service, coming finally to the the altar call and the closing benediction. There will never be a more reverent or meaningful Sunday morning service than that one; or a daughter more determined that nothing was going to keep her father from church on Sunday.

After Martha's call and my "Suck it up, you wimp" pep talk, I was out of ICU in 24 hours. And notes like this one from the unflappable ladies of the Tuesday Club gave me a last little push. I thought I was having a rough time in ICU but the ladies of the Tuesday Club let me know things were rough all over.

58

Tuesday, March 27, 1990

Buffalo,

I couldn't resist taking this card along to Tuesday Club this afternoon for all to sign. You will note some signatures of people you never heard of—I told them that didn't matter, that it wouldn't upset you to know that a roomful of 30 women were all thinking about you, whether you know them or not!

It was the usual hilarious meeting—Mrs.____went sound asleep in the middle of the program, and the hostess was sick in the bedroom with bronchitis and never appeared. Jane was the co-hostess in charge of refreshments but didn't know it until yesterday but did an admirable job of pulling Christmas fudge out of the freezer...You know we're all behind you—and with the entire Tuesday Club on your side, that is pretty formidable.

Love from all the Kimbroughs

There was so much energy and love coming to me from everywhere. Genie once said in a TV interview that she believed energy can be transferred to another person. She certainly proved that in caring for me. She and the family really cared for me *hands* on and I could actually feel the strength and energy in their touch. It's not easy for a big guy like myself to allow others to care for him in such a personal way––no privacy, no machismo, no Brut, just a heap of quivering, shivering, naked, grossly swollen flesh.

It's not easy to give that kind of care, and it's not easy to accept it. But in allowing myself to be cared for in this most intimate way I made a stunning discovery. I found that I was not exposing my helplessness but rather allowing all of us to explore the richness of our human condition at both ends of Give and Take. Even at the hard rock bottom of need, there is treasure to be mined.

We need to extend our concept of the human condition to encompass not just the strong, the healthy, the best and the brightest but those at the other end, as well. Why should we feel a distinct sadness at the thought of illness and old age but not at the *years* we spend taking care of the all-consuming demands of our infants and young children? All are part of life.

Family and teammates learned one important truth. Our most profound insights into our humanity come from helping one another. To allow ourselves to be human enough to feel and share with someone else, is to enlarge our understanding of what it means to be a human being. It is empowering. It is elevating. It is the ultimate bonding experience.

Once you have been transformed by this overwhelming sense of your own humanity, winning your battles becomes secondary. The indomitable victory is in this discovery of *self*, in the largest possible sense of that word.

What we were learning from each other was more precious than a guaranteed warranty on life because what we were learning guaranteed that we would enjoy the life we had to the hilt.

Neither my big sister, family, nor my team would cut me any slack or let me off the hook while I was fighting off the effects of IL-2.

My cousin Jenny acknowledged that the going was rough but she also refused to throw in the towel. My team was more confident than I was that there was still some fight left in me. And Jenny sent me a secret weapon. It worked.

May 9, 1990

Dear Bob,

You have been real sick. Everybody says. We are so sorry and would do anything to help you if we could, but this seems to be very much like Lindbergh's flight over the Atlantic—all alone with barely enough light to read his maps, not much food, and not feeling too great. But Lord!—that moment when he saw the sun shining off the coast of France and realized that he'd made it!

My friend wanted me to go with her to see the movie Glory. *I told her to save her popcorn, that it was being enacted in awful living color with real live heroes in Duke hospital even as we spoke. Bob Stone carries our regiment flag, I said, and we don't look for it to fall, or touch ground. It IS hanging pretty low but that is on account of the rough terrain and hazardous footing. But the boy is brave and has good shoes. I am plenty worried, but you can keep your white hanky in your breast pocket, I said to her.*

Bob, do you remember when all the Stone Boys had to special order their shoes (Size 15 up) from Winston-Salem and the clerk would call long distance to Stoneville with the message: TELL THE STONE BOYS THEIR SHOES ARE HERE. Well, I think you got your shoes out of the same lot as the rest of those big, gallant men we so loved. Yes, Bob Stone your shoes are here and they aren't easy to fill. Know it.

Tom Robinson talked to one of his doctor friends the other day and he said, if he can stand the

61

treatment, live through this, he's got it licked. Amen.

I am in constant contact with the Schwinn people. We have another contender who broke out of the pack like a Buffalo. He looked real good briefly, then faded. The red bike was an eye-catcher but it turned out he didn't believe in anything—not red bikes, not God, not nothing. He got cured of his cancer but lost the whole point of the game. He didn't think there was a point or really much of a game. Well you better believe that our outfitters at Schwinn think there is a point. That's why they advertise in Boys Life*. So it looks like the Buffaloes are trampling all competition by simply being mulish which they have learned from hanging out and being sociable.*

Anyway, the Schwinn people wanted to know if we wanted red metallic paint on the bike—flame, they called it. I told them we wanted it to be REAL RED and they are working on it. Thus far the score is in your favor. You have the most points earned and there's no doubt about it. I can almost feel that pedal power under foot. Can you?

Bob I want so badly to help you. I sat down last night and thought what would I want if I were up against it. And like magic I was seven years old and sitting on a creek bank, feeling cool moss like velvet under my bare feet. I was a strong and mighty brave, I could see in the dark, I wasn't afraid. Because in my hand I had a secret weapon. Only me and God knew about it. I pass it along to you.

Enclosed is what every stalwart Prayer Warrior needs: a shotgun shell loaded with Scripture. Not just any Scripture but the verses you have particularly asked us to read. Every verse is packed in this shell and ready to be fired. I put it on a rawhide thong taken from the hide of one mean buffalo. The mere sight of this super-charged shell around your neck is enough to make those C-Cells run. This is heavy duty power. This is magic. This is the power of Our Lord in a magnum shell.

Keep campaigning hard. Go with God and give 'em hell, Bob.

Love, Jenny

No doubt about it, God in a magnum shotgun shell definitely gives you the edge on the competition. "Put it around my neck," I instructed Genie. She slipped the rawhide tong over my head. I thought of all the Scripture verses I had asked the team to read along with me. Most of those verses were about hope and love. I believe God shows His love for us through our friends. A friend is His way of sending His love to us in way we can touch and feel and respond to. A way of loving God right back. My new amulet was evidence of that love.

When I checked out of Duke three days later they wanted to take me out in a wheelchair. Is this the way a warrior goes home? Is this the way a *Buffalo* leaves the field? With Genie on one side and my sister Martha on the other, they half dragged, half-carried me out of the hospital and loaded me into the back seat of the car. "Where next?" Genie joked, turning the nose of the car toward the mountains.

Wobbly as a spring colt, covered in skin rash, I still felt like shouting. I swear I could almost see the sun shining off the

63

coast of France after an exhausting perilous flight. I had made it! Round number two of IL-2 treatment was now in the record books, one more to go.

"How about a pit stop for a burger and shake?" I wheedled. Forbidden food, I knew, but the smell of a fast food hamburger was exactly what was needed to dissipate the overpowering odor of Eau de ICU that still clung to me. I watched the hospital recede in the distance as we headed home.

I suddenly felt a surge of pure happiness. I was going home—and one more thing. The Buffaloes were way out ahead in the race for the red bike.

NINE

Getting Beat Up By Experts

Anyone who has been through it will tell you that the low times during any long-term battle is when one skirmish is over and you are suspended in time, waiting for the next one. This is when you bottom-out, waiting through excruciating long weeks for latest test results. Are the tumors shrinking? Is the medication effective? Can you muster enough strength to go one more round?

IL-2 was like getting beat up by experts. It required all my skill at visualization to even imagine getting through the next treatments.

Genie was heroically (and single-handedly) nourishing me back to health with tempting low-fat, vitamin-loaded, easy-to-digest food. I would come to the table, eat a few bites and become so exhausted that I had to go back to bed. Then I'd get up again and eat a few more bites. It was a long slow road, getting my weight back and recovering from the toxic effects of my treatment. Getting myself back in good physical condition was as important as what they were doing for me at Duke. The most advanced, aggressive therapy in the world wouldn't be worth a hill of beans if I wasn't in shape to take my chances with it.

That spring and summer, we were living on the edge. It seemed we were always *waiting*—sweating out a new series of tests so we could see how the cancer was progressing—or *not* progressing, as we desperately hoped.

Doubts cruise sluggishly down an endless Amazon on that dark continent of the big D. You have faced Mortality with such regularity that you can count on one thing. Now no one blinks. Death is no longer that dream you can't quite remember; it is always there, in your peripheral field of vision. Death happens all around you. With every return visit to Duke came the news of a friend on the Jordan Ward who didn't make it. You steeled yourself for that fleeting look of pain when you asked about someone, or got a phone call or note from a member of their family. Many of those I have mentioned in this book like Egil Hagen and Suzanne Lewis did not outlive their disease. But, I believe, they did outlive their fear of the disease. And by squarely facing this fear, they were able to see the world spread out around them from a fresh perspective. We have learned much from each other.

And from that fresh perspective I wonder if we do not fear life as much as we fear death. We come to fear life when we are told that we're fresh out of time—time to get to know our kids, time to reconnect to old friends and make new ones, time to appreciate our marriage. We do love to proscrastinate. Suddenly we find that we no longer have "tomorrow and tomorrow and tomorrow" to make good on those promises we made to ourselves. For too many of us, our own lives are like that book we really meant to read, but never got around to. Facing our mortality can be the bleak prospect of a black hole at the core of our existence, created by a wanton depletion of self and energy. A cluttered, directionless, rudderless life coupled with a compressed time frame may be what we actually fear as much as we fear death. Often it takes illness or an inescapable challenge to expose this crucial deficiency in our lives. It is *that* death we fear and must reckon with, as much as physical death.

This brings me unerringly to the subject of porch swings and gliders. I spent many hours that summer I was regaining my strength in one or the other. I discovered that my "ninetysomething" Uncle Charlie was right. You get a much better slant on things from a porch swing. The rump view of life. A swing hanging from a well-oiled chain, or an old-fashioned glider, like we had on our screened porch in Charlotte, not only loosens you up, but everyone else around you, as well. A son throws his legs over the arms of a nearby rocker and opens up about his life, a friend drops by with a seed catalog and shares her thoughts on rhododendrons and old age (both plant and friend handle it admirably). And before you know it, you find yourself being healed, spiritually if not physically.

Call it a team, a community or just hanging out with the guys and gals—but allowing yourself to become part of a larger part is miraculously restorative. At Duke hospital, a fellow in ICU is a big deal. He is stripped, examined, plugged into weird machines, monitored 24 hours a day around the clock.

But here on my porch in my wonderful swing, life flows around me, blessedly without undue notice or alarm...I doze off with the sound of Genie talking to our dog Maggie as they plant annuals, a tractor across the way strains up the hill, a couple of weekenders call to each other while picking blackberries down by the creek. The cool deep smell of summer is everywhere. I awaken with a throw tossed over me, soup left warming on the stove. My needs are seen to sensibly and routinely, just as Maggie's are—water in her bowl, food in her dish, a dry place in a sudden shower. The flow of life happening all around can be wonderfully healing. We only need to let it happen, to allow time for it to happen.

The question of death was one Genie and I had already faced —for me, while in ICU or watching an IV drip its relentless, near-lethal dose into my veins. And for Genie, while she waited, watching the seasons change from winter to spring then to summer from the window of our room on the Jordan Ward. For both of us the next searching question became would I have a life left to live after IL-2—after those C-cells had exploded like a Devil's puffball, carrying deadly spores throughout my body.

Giving in to these very natural feelings of anxiety was exactly what I could not afford to do. Disease feeds on despair. Negative feelings can render the immune system's defenses useless. A

67

positive attitude is not only a plus, it can be the whole ball game.

Any protracted crisis situation imposes its own strict discipline. In living with crisis, day in and day out, you find yourself becoming more reflective. Crisis changes your perspective, forces you to want to change stressful, hurtful relationships. This is good. What you must avoid is playing over and over again those same old tapes of guilt and frustration we carry around with us—playing backup guitar to the What-Might-Have-Beens. Endless examining of unfulfilled or unresolved relationships with a parent, a child, or even a business associate can cripple a recovery program.

I needed my team as never before. Waiting can be a team effort. Everyone can dress out. Everyone can play. In a brief letter I leveled with the Buffaloes. I tried to give them a sense of my emotional turbulence—the joy of having made it through my treatment, by the skin of my teeth, and the painful uncertainty of the weeks that lay ahead.

May 17, 1990

Dear Team,

There is no place like home! Having spent the last three and a half weeks in the hospital, you can imagine what it is like to get to your own bed, eat home-cooked food and smell fresh air. It's wonderful!

First let me thank you again for your cards, letters, jokes, pictures, and prayers that you sent to pull the team through. We made it, Gang, with flying colors, but with some difficulty at the end. Jenny's letter referred to me as a sick man. This was because I had to go to intensive care for three days at the end of my IL-2 treatment. I was in la-la land—some funny stories to tell here. At any rate, we are now ready to get back in shape for the next round.

Secondly, you need to know that Genie, Tyler, and Marion did an outstanding job of coaching. You team members were terrific support. I am a lucky man!

Q. When will you know if IL-2 Plus LAK did the job?
A. We'll have answers sometime in June.
Q. What will be the next step?
A. Not sure, but will drop you a postcard when certain.
Q. What is the South Carolina state fossil?
A. Strom Thurmond - courtesy of Charlotte Observer.
Q. Is it mandatory to use the Buffalo bumper sticker?
A. No. Avid team member from VA printed 500 with the following suggestions:
  1. Use as bumper sticker to invite discussion on how one family is fighting cancer.
  2. Keep for your next scavenger hunt.
  3. Perfect for 1990 time capsule.
Q. What is the best medicine I've had?
A. Laughter is the best medicine.

We will be renewing our physical strength and renewing our spiritual strength in the mountains, but wish you all a lovely spring, happy graduations, wonderful weddings, and much joy, love, and peace.

Love, Bob
Romans 8:28

Sometimes not knowing what's ahead is a real blessing. But Genie and I knew what was ahead of us in the second and third rounds of therapy. We faced it with equal parts of dread and hope. The minute by minute brinkmanship we had gone through in ICU still hung over us like a threatening cloud. The test results were so encouraging it was difficult not to take the money and run, hoping that the residual IL-2 in my body would finish a mop-up campaign on those few remaining cancer cells. Aggressive therapy takes a real commitment on the part of the patient. It takes some real hard coaching to keep yourself mentally in shape for the road ahead—especially when you know what's down that road.

We never felt more keenly the isolation and separation that serious illness imposes. Even the huge enduring mountains of the Blue Ridge seemed to close about us, blocking out everything beyond, so there was only the sound of our own heart beating. And a God who had not abandoned us.

TEN

No Ordinary Ham

My team, the Buffaloes, wouldn't let me call it quits with IL-2. They wanted the whole series. They wanted that red bike, in full dress with raccoon tails. The pepper and coaching from the bench echoed throughout the Carolina mountains.

One curious shopper at a mall noted one of our Buffalo bumper stickers. "Is that a pro team or semi-pro?"

"Definitely pro," a fiesty Buffalo fired back.

The team had learned a lot. Messages reeled off the machine, my mailbox was stuffed with notes and cards which in turn were stuffed with cartoons, snapshots, and enough craziness to make me wonder if I were still hallucinating.

The Buffaloes certainly had their share of journal writers, letter writers, screen writers, sky writers. It is a sheer impossibility to single out every noteworthy letter. This book would be as weighty as *The Rise and Fall of Western Civilization*. But just a whiff is all it takes to tell you how rich the stew is!

It was not any *one* letter that made the difference, it was the weight, the heft of all those letters behind me that got me through. My sister Martha is a busy first grade teacher. She was also very worried about her kid brother. With little time to indulge creative flights of fancy, Martha opted for *constancy*. Each day's mail brought a card, a note, a letter, a small gift. Each day's mail for seven long months. Her contribution to the team was not one brilliant *tour de force* but her faithful bearing with another human being, day in and day out.

Phil Hazel sure didn't write me every day but when he did, he got my attention. Phil was czar of two small municipal airports by day, closet screen-writer by night. His screen treatment of his projected feature-length film was either forgettable or unforgettable—you choose!

September 1, 1990

Yo, Mountain Buffalo,

Each day we await news from the world capitals: Washington, Paris, London, Baghdad, Amman, Riyahd and the Blue Ridge. I have a swap to propose for Buffalo negotiators––the oil price can go wherever, the Iraqis get out of Kuwait and C gets out of Buffalo territory, starting with an immediate withdrawal from all of the invaded areas. This will make red bicycles mandatory for all of us.

The reason for moving to the mountains is bureaucratic. The post office will not allow General Delivery mail after 30 days so you had to get a P.O. Box so you might as well move. I like it. The only logical conclusion to reach.

How about a film like "The Bear?" Picture this:

Scene I: A young buffalo is seen roaming the streets of an urban center. Young buffalo is constantly getting stung by bees, stepping on rattlesnakes, falling down cliffs and experiencing other travails because he repeatedly tries to live life to the fullest.

Scene II: A maturing but playful buffalo finds mate and begins family in new locale. Spends a lot of time hunting for the best place to graze, chasing other buffalos away, showing new buffalo calves where not to step and leading less fortunate wildlife to fresher water, greener grass and bluer skies.

Scene III: Buffalo watches as calves grow into buffaloes, too. Buffalo missus shows creative side. Green grass becomes harder to find, pressure rises to find fresh water, buffalo internalizes—bad for any buffalo. Suddenly, while buffalo internalizing, Indians (merely a metaphor, not a reflection on any ethnic group) appear and buffalo catches a few arrows. Buffalo bellows. Other buffaloes circle wounded buffalo. Other wildlife, previously shown greener grass, fresher water, bluer skies by buffalo return to circle around buffalo and drive Indians off. Buffalo nurses wounds. It is not easy but buffalo healing.

Scene IV: Buffalo stands on mountain top. Cool stream runs below. Water is fresh and plentiful. Grass has never been greener. Sky never bluer. Indians not a problem. Buffalo gets a post office box.

Your faith, determination and example offers us as much support as we offer you. You continue as a model for the efficient use of resources. You always put back more than you use. We think about you every day.

Love, The Hazels

I attribute the startling diversity of the Buffalo Letters to a single factor. Ham. Country cured in the heart of the Southland, liberally salted with humor, rubbed good with pepper and aged to perfection. The result produces a ham that could tempt even a listless appetite like mine. The ham produced from one of our Buffaloes, was tender, richly flavored, and, above all, didn't shrink away to a memory in the frying pan.

The test results of the first IL-2 Plus LAK gave us the momentum we needed for that next round of treatment. I couldn't wait to tell the team.

June 16, 1990

Dear Team,

LET THE GAMES CONTINUE!
Score
THE BUFFALOES 98   CANCER 2

The word from our doctor at Duke is "That we're on the right track." We were very happy to get this news and to learn that the IL-2 Plus LAK cell treatment has caused the tumors on my lungs to shrink. We go back for tests on July 2, 3, and 9. On July 16th, the Team suits up again for our second offensive push which will end August 3. Genie, Tyler, Marion and I are very grateful to you for your efforts to date, and ask that you stay in training and gear up for this next push. Your support means SO much.

To say that we are enjoying the mountains would be an understatement. Genie has had a wonderful time in her flower garden and has had a little time for her painting. Marion has a part-time job and has been doing a great deal of hiking with our new ten month old puppy, Maggie. Tyler continues to work for Northwestern Mutual Life in Charlotte and joins us on the weekends. I continue to gain my strength and enjoy Genie's cooking. We are all excited about a family fishing trip to Montana the last week in June. Look out trout!

I hope that your spring has been a good one and that your Summer plans are taking shape. We have enjoyed hearing from you and being brought up-to-date on the news from you and your families. You are good friends.

A bit of British humor:
Johnny (to his mother): "I don't want to go to school today.
Mother: "Why not? You haven't been for five days."
Johnny: "The girls tease me, the boys bully me, the staff are unsympathetic."
Mother: "Pull your socks up, Johnny, you're 49 now and the headmaster."

Word from my cousin Jenny is that the Buffaloes are still trampling the competition, and things continue to look good for winning the red Schwinn bike! I'm wearing my secret weapon she sent and campaigning hard. Your continued support and prayers mean MORE *than you know. We continue to feel very blessed.*

Love, Bob
Exodus 23:25

P.S. Norman Cousin's book, Head First: The Biology of Hope *is on the best seller list. Read it and give it to a friend.*

WHERE THE BUFFALOES ROAM

My cousin Jenny launched an all-out campaign to edge me back into the fray. She warned me of competition for the Real Red bike. Jenny's fictional but very correct Mr. Tripp Winn let us know that he wasn't in the business of *giving* out his bikes. No sir, a guy had to win his bike fair and square. And that Real Red paint color on my bike was giving him a fit.

July 11, 1990

Dear Bob,

I know you are getting ready for another big push in the games. Word is that the bumper stickers are going like hot cakes in Africa. Stan is hot and hungry and speaking French like a pro. We are all preparing to suit up in case you need us to come off the bench and throw a few key blocks for you. While you were off fishing I've had my trials down here. Tripp Winn from the Schwinn Company called the other day. It went like this:

Ms. Stone-Humphries, Winn with Schwinn here. I've the latest communication from our Bob Stone in hand. What a pip of a fight! We've all been following it. You can be sure all of us here are readying for another massive push *to get Bob Stone through his ordeal and back to—wherever. I believe he topped his own personal best in this last round of the games. I thought we'd lost him right at the last. He's recovering at home?*

Nope, Montana. Where the you-know-what roam and seldom is heard a discouraging word.

To be Sure. I must say our man, Bob Stone is not easy to keep track of. It certainly hasn't been easy to keep on top of his progress toward Total Wellness. You spoke of his flying all alone over the Atlantic, of magnum shotgun shells and Indian warriors, carrying the regimental colors into the face of unbelievable odds—the boy has good shoes? Gracious, even the outfitters of Stone expeditionary forces are awed! Where is Bob Stone we ask daily—in the air, on land or at sea?

Yep. Now about the bike, Have you got the bugs worked out of that Real Red? What's the delay in sending down the latest paint samples?

Let's talk about that Real Red you requested. We really can't spray on the final color until we know exactly who *has won the machine. I mean fair is fair. An open competition, right? I mean that's what the Schwinn Company has built its reputation on—a fair race among fair-minded boys. We like to think of all of our boys as being physically strong, mentally fit, morally straight— in a word, Ms. Stone-Humphries,* all *our boys have good shoes!*

Tripp, don't make me go over to a competitor. I saw a nifty mountain bike in the L.L. Bean catalog.

You can't be serious! L.L. Bean makes GUM SHOES AND DUFFLES. Schwinn makes cycling machines. I broach the matter of the paint as a simple practicality. What if we go with Real Red and the winner were disappointed? Bob won't be disappointed. It's free. What I'm getting to is simply this. Your Bob Stone may not win the bike. Someone else could come on strong and take it.

And what if he or she did not want a Real Red bike. What if their taste ran to a more whimsical color? Our Giverny Blue has been a runaway hit this season.

Tripp, no one whose taste runs to Giverny Blue has a chance of winning your bike. Know it. Besides no one is coming on stronger than our man, Bob.

He could lag in the home stretch—the thought gives me chilblains. He could have equipment failure.

He's already had *equipment failure. Didn't faze him. He blew a tire in the homestretch this last time in Duke. Genie did have to get down off the handlebars but that was the extent of the damage control. Let's see one of your Giverny Blue crowd match that. Besides red is the color we want. Red is the color of courage. As in* Red Badge of... *Red is the Fun Color. Look at fire engines, electric trains, wagons, trikes, sports cars.*

Enough, enough, Ms. Stone-Humphries. I'm weary of the debate. I'll give the shop the go ahead on Real Red.

Good. Now we can go on to the next thing on the list.

What's that?

Squirrel tails.

Squirrel tails?

No Ordinary Ham

For the handlebars. What kind of winter are they predicting up there, Tripp? We like 'em bushy.

KEEP YOUR EYE ON THE PRIZE, BOB STONE!!!

Love, Jenny

A wild embroglio ensued. The Real Red bike, which some had thought was a gimmick or a metaphor of Jenny's imagination was real! David Grimes, my prayer buddy, called Jenny to get this straight. "You know at first I thought the red bike was a gimmick––just to get Bob going. But now with all this talk about real red paint—is there really a bike, Jenny?"

"It's a Schwinn," Jenny reminded David.

"It is real then. There really *is* a bike. I mean it's real!" Some of the guys in the group thought it might be just PR. But it's not, right? It's real!" David began to sound like a kid who aches for a racy red bike.

"It's real all right. Real red."

Real became the operative word. It set off more stunting and double loops than even my high-flying friend Phil Hazel could follow. Phil circled back to give me a unforgettable liftoff for my final battle with the protocol at Duke. As usual he saw possibilities the rest of us had missed:

> *Pam and I would like to act as attorney and agent when you write your memoirs. We think it has real appeal to the masses and we think we can get you a terrific deal with Touchstone Pictures. There has been some preliminary discussion in Hollywood on casting. It looks like Signourney Weaver is set for Genie, with either Tom Cruise in lifts or Alan Alda as the Buffalo. ...T-Shirts, coffee mugs and caps look to generate some real good cash flow. McDonalds is concepting a Buffalo-burger in test markets and they see it as a tie-in with Teenage Mutant Ninja*

WHERE THE BUFFALOES ROAM

IL-2 Plus LAK. THE POSSIBILITIES ARE ENDLESS.
Aaaahhh, but you already knew that.

(letter from Phil Hazel, Statesville, N.C.)

Excitement escalated. The Buffaloes didn't want blood—they wanted red paint. And more. The team didn't want any late comers coming on strong and stealing our bike in the homestretch. Letters poured in. They offered advice. They pooh-poohed any contender with a preference for Giverny blue. Even the staid Davidson Journal gave late-breaking coverage on our challenge race for the mountain bike.

Friends reported that the Buffalo bumper sticker was becoming a very trendy item, sported on only the best bumpers. The stickers were traded and sought after as authoritative proof of team membership.

My nephew, Stan, a teacher with the Peace Corps, was director of our most distant Buffalo outpost—in Benin, West Africa. Stan sent me a photo of his youthful Natitingou team displaying our bumper sticker. That picture earned a prominent place in our official Buffalo team program, as proof the team concept can translate itself between continents, between countries, between languages, between human hearts. And nothing is lost in the translation. Everyone understands a *team*.

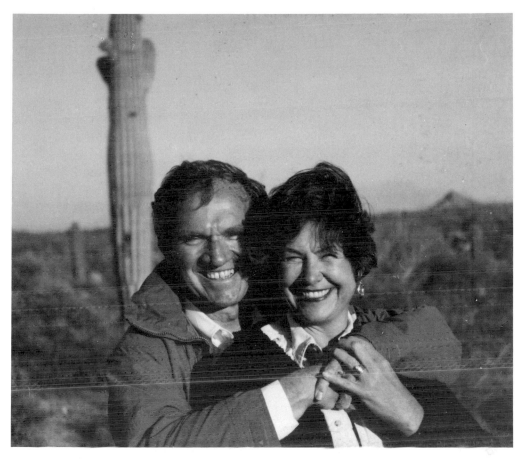

Me and my gal

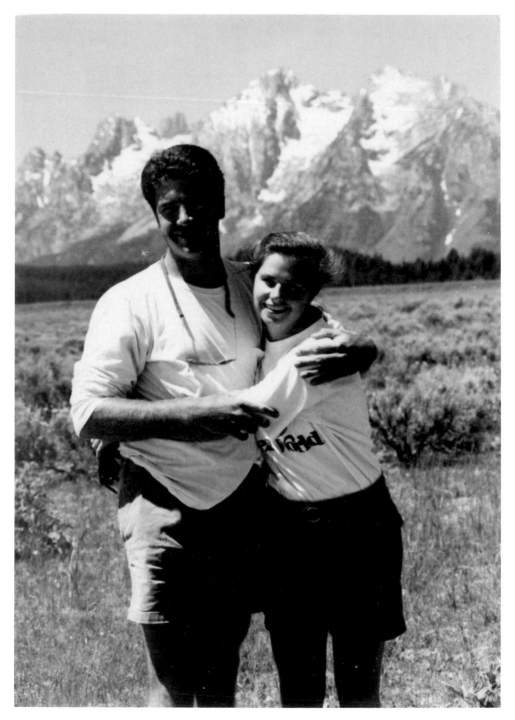

Tyler and Marion Stone—our two

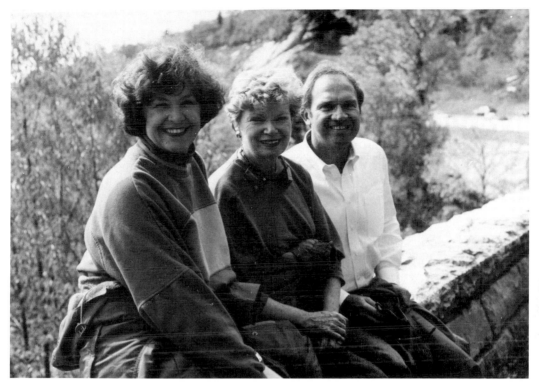

Genie and me, with my sister Martha—Autumn on the Blue Ridge Parkway

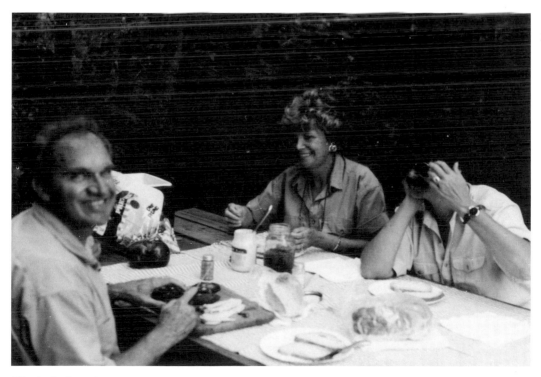

We picnic along the way.

Jenny Stone Humphries
without typewriter

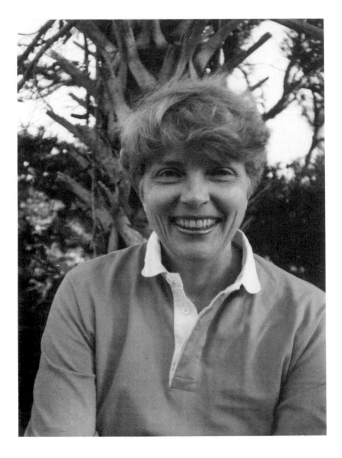

My sister Martha with her first
grade class of banner artists.
They livened up the decor.

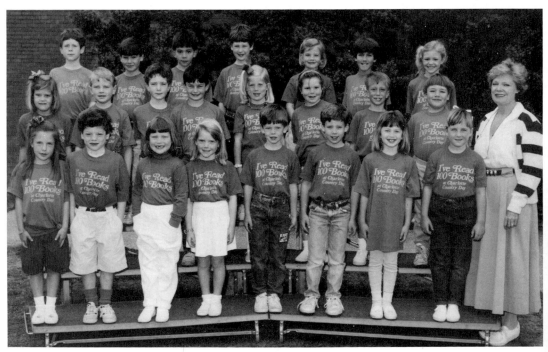

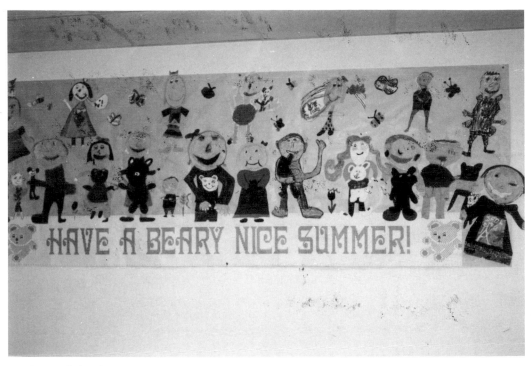

Here's one of their banners.

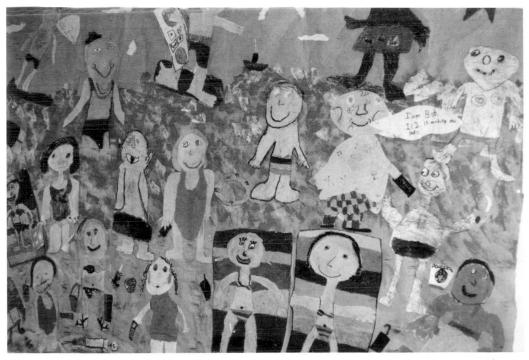

Not bad at murals, either! Note the guy saying, "I am Bob. IL-2 is making me fat!!"   And how.

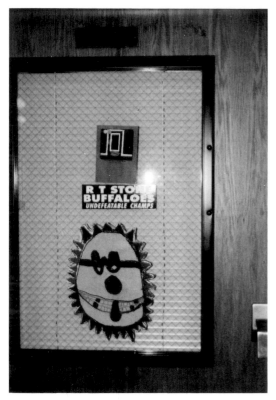

The door to my room on the Jordan Ward
at the Duke Comprehensive Cancer Center

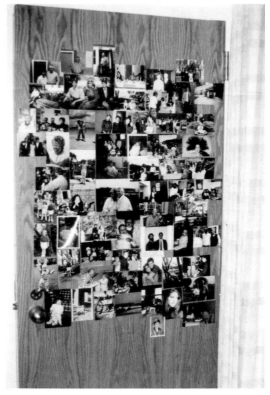

The bed with a view

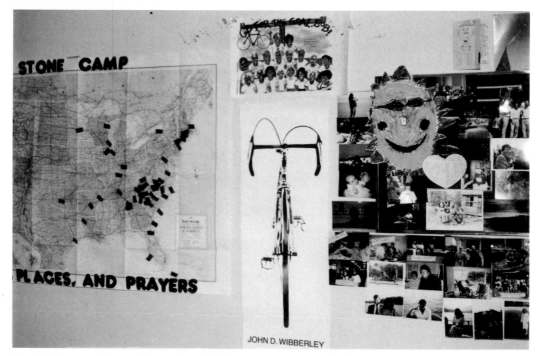

People, Places and Prayers Map—where Buffaloes roam! Note picture of bike to keep me focused.

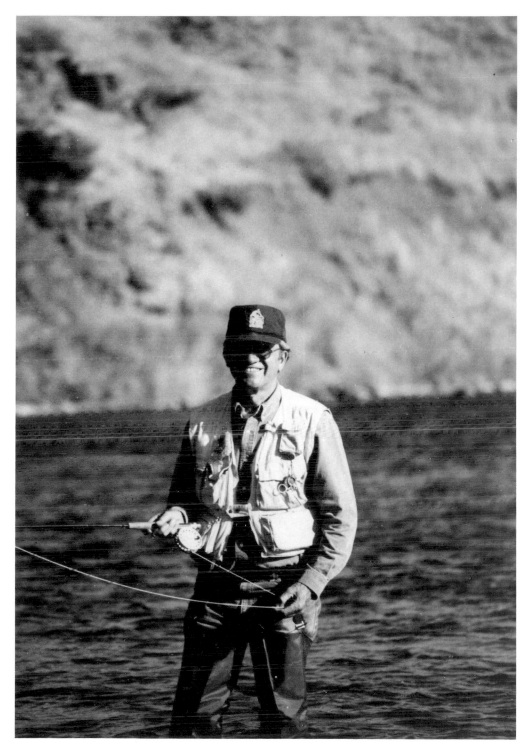

Casting for Big Daddy in Montana

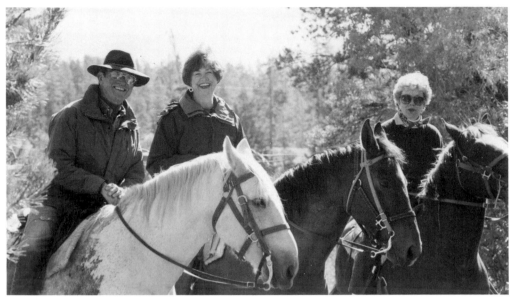

Genie and me with Jane Avinger

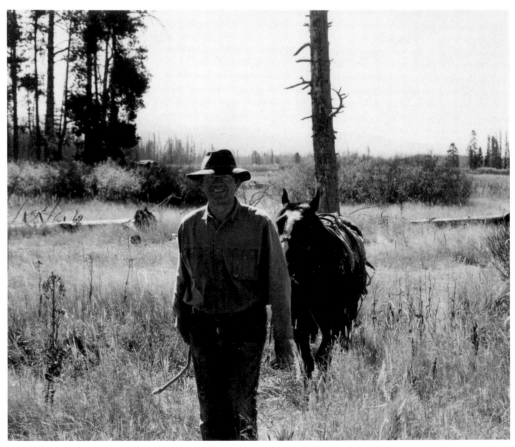

Out in the field, tracking buffalo

Genie, with her brother Tom
Stallworth and his family

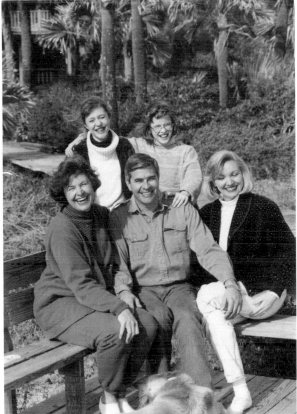

Genie at the Outer Banks

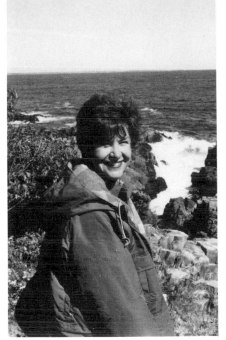

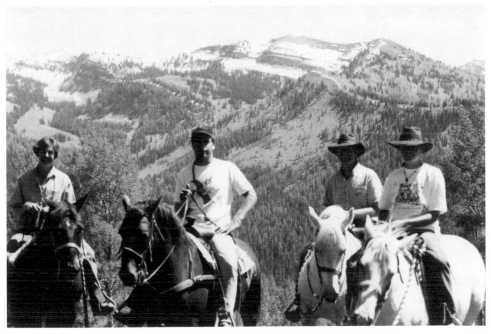

Me and the family—four desperadoes

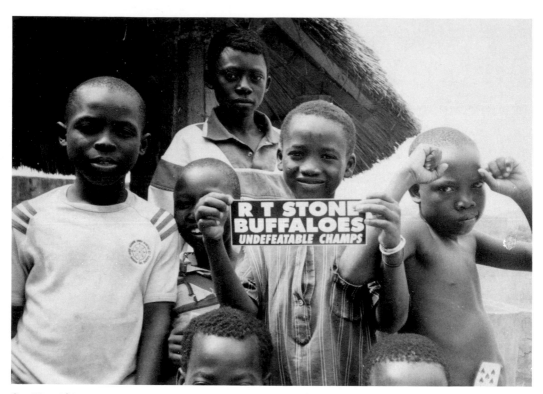

Our West African team

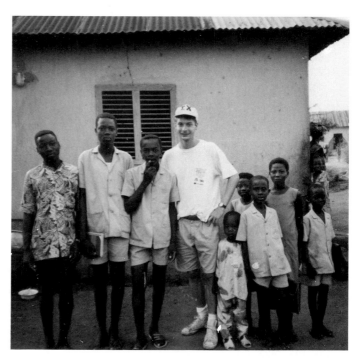

Stan Humphries at our most distant outpost in Natitingou with more Buffaloes!

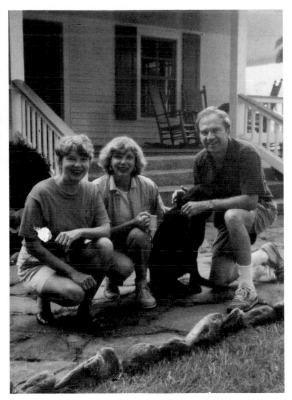

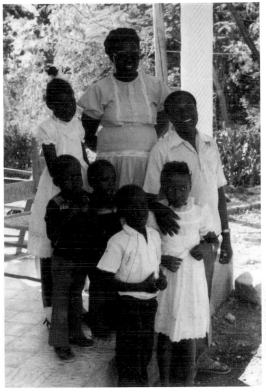

Jenny and her twin Betty visiting us in the mountains just before the IL-2 wars

The Reverend Michael Morisset and family, of Haiti. His church members prayed for me around the clock, twenty-four hours a day.

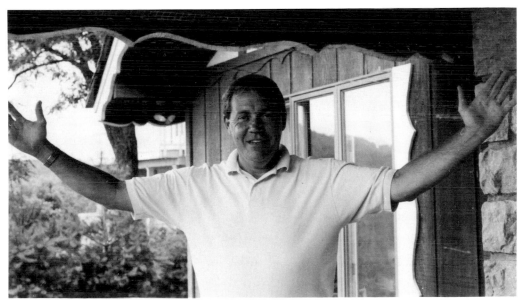

Phil Hazel, our closet screenwriter, concepting his latest project—BIG!

Our couples study group. Major players (left to right): Doug MacNeil, Janey MacNeil, Larry Christie, Jean Winje-Christie (Jean staked out the buffalo postcard for the team), Nancy Kelley, Genie Stone, Pete Kelley.

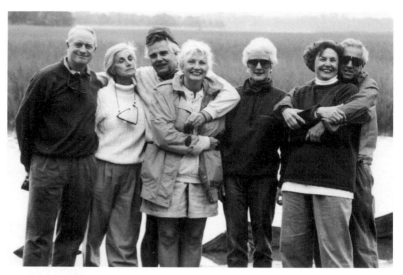

Snow, Dylan and Maggie

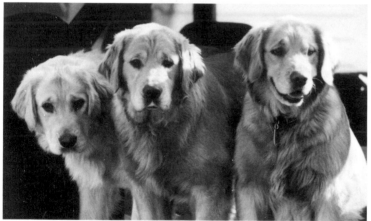

Suzanne Lewis with Genie. Suzanne started her own team.

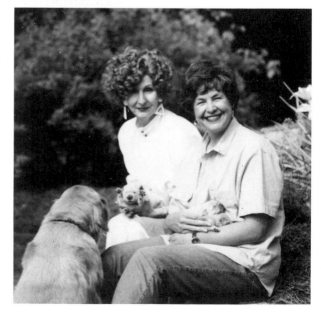

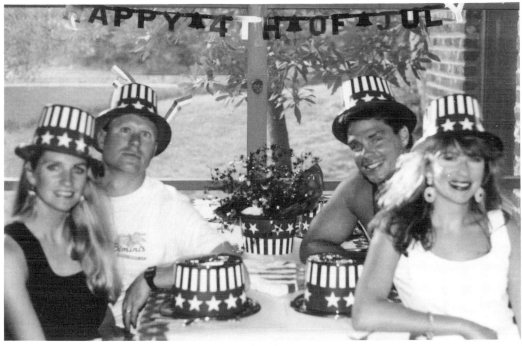

Bonnie and Bruce, Johnny and Donna: my sister's kids with spouses. Party animals!

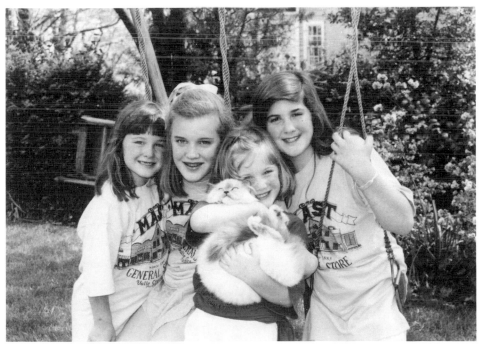

The lovely Hassenfelt girls from next door in Greensboro

Surveying fallout after the move from Greensboro to the mountains. Does your garage look like this?

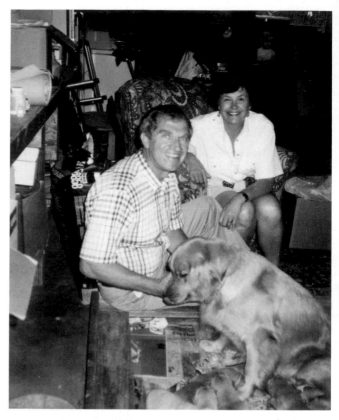

Plotting team strategy for final leg of race for bike

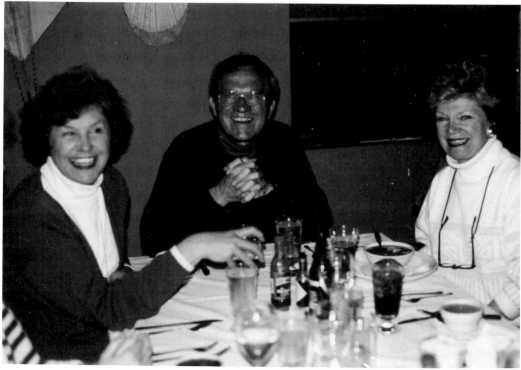

At Genie's training table

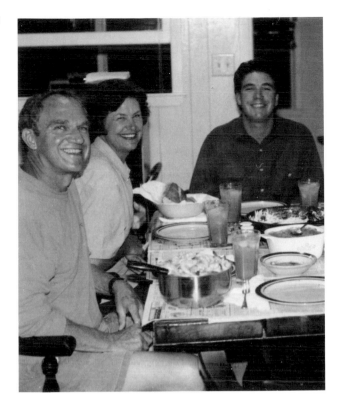

A boy and his bike.
What a Christmas!

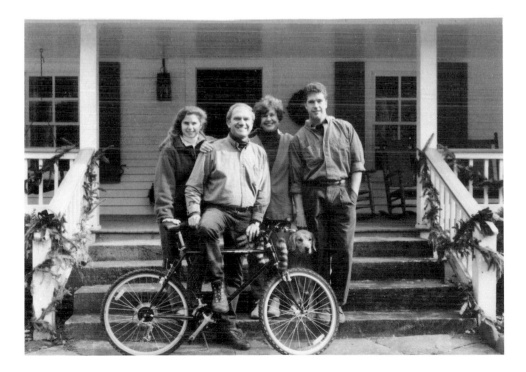

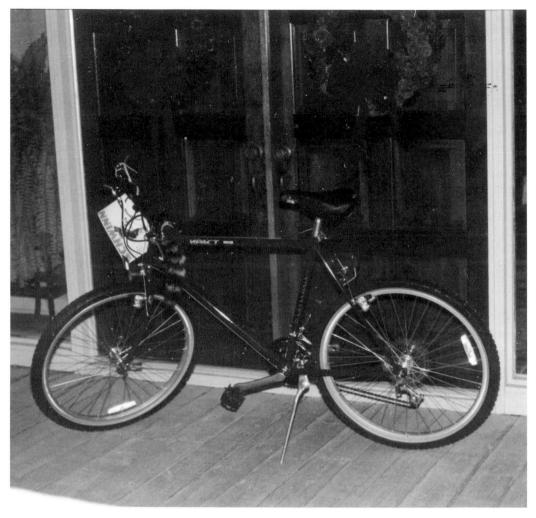

The prize worth winning—MTB # REAL RED—with raccoon tails

ELEVEN

Going For the Win

Genie thought we needed a change of venue. Boys, let's move this tired herd to Montana! So off we trekked to the home of the big buffaloes, to see cactus and purple sage, to see if the trout would rise to our flies. We even found four horses who were very forgiving of four novice cowpokes.

We returned from the land of the Big Sky saddle sore, with our limit of trout, and renewed. We checked back into Duke for another scan. The news was too good to keep!

August 30, 1990

Dear Team,

I hope this letter finds you in good health with many happy and interesting memories from your summer experience. We have heard about the wonderful weddings, trips to camp, the beach, the mountains, and the fishing outings. Our trip to Montana could not have been more fun, and it looks as though Tyler and I have been joined by two other fly-fishing enthusiasts. Genie and Marion became "pros" with their fly-rods and were catching rainbows in Montana with the best of them!

BUFFALOES - 99 CANCER - 1

Gooo Buffaloes! We're doing it TEAM! I have just returned from Duke and a CAT scan. My doctor reports that the cancer continues to diminish and that I can count on Game 3 sometime in October. Game 2 was a tough one, and I feel I must tell you something because it's very important to the team concept.

In my quest for the Real Red Bike Jenny writes about in her letter, I became overzealous and ended up in Duke's intensive care unit again. When they wheeled me in, I was very, very weak. It was a difficult time, and I prayed for strength to get through the next couple of hours. I began thinking about my family, each of you, your calls, your letters and cards, the jokes, the books, the wonderful photographs you have sent and then I had the thought—Stone, you wimp! Suck it up, the Buffaloes are pulling for you and you need to get tough—I was out of there in a day and a half! My point is this—I could not have done it without family and friends—the team concept works!

The other news I wish to share with you is that Genie and I have decided to move to the mountains. We had planned to retire there someday, but my medical situation has just moved it up a few years. It's sad to leave our friends in Greensboro, but we plan on keeping close ties and counting on you to come see us in the mountains.

I think that October 7th will be the day I return to Duke. If you have a chance, say a little prayer

Going For the Win

*for us. It means so much. Genie, Tyler and
Marion join me in sending you our love.*

*Love Bob
"I always thank God for you..."
I Corinthians 1:4 NIV*

My third and final IL-2 Plus LAK treatment got underway in
October. It proved to be a poltergeist, unleashing a devastating
cumulative effect built up over previous treatments. It was like
food poisoning, dysentery, and hell all rolled into one two-week,
non-refundable package.

One side-effect of IL-2 was terrific edema. My body became
swollen and grotesquely distended with fluid. I hardly recognized
the face I saw in the mirror. That was the only humorous moment
in a grim siege. That gross, fat face surely wasn't mine, I decided.
Someone had snatched my body! I reeled the telephone in, and
put through a Mayday to Genie in her hotel room. "Come on over
here and see what they've done to me," I rasped, slamming the
receiver down. Then I dialed my sister Martha. Surely my big sister
could do something about this alien who had taken possession of
her brother's body. "You won't believe what they've done,
Martha. You won't recognize me. I'm ruined!"

As my third treatment progressed, unendurable pain
gripped my fingers and extremities in a vise that even morphine
couldn't ease. A toxic reaction from the IL-2 in my body. Groggy
and heavily sedated, I woke up one afternoon with a nurse
disconnecting my IV apparatus. "Is it over?" I whispered.

"For you it is."

Our final game had been called with three days left to go
with IL-2. Did I get enough of the treatment to assure that the job
was done? Or was all the pain and sickness for nothing? We
wouldn't know for four weeks.

During that time, I also had a puzzling dream. I saw a
industrial-sized vacuum sweeper rolling over my body. This huge

sweeper was relentlessly sucking up billions of cancer cells, as fine as grains of sand and as numerous. Was my body telling me that the job was too big, there were more cancer cells than could possibly be vacuumed up? Was my body telling me that all the jokes, visualization, positive attitude and prayers still could not balance the terrible odds? Or was my body giving me the good news by showing me it had the cancer cells under control? Which? That's what I didn't know.

My doctor, Philip Walther, looked like a kid who was having trouble waiting his turn. He rammed my latest X-rays into the viewing box. "Bob, it's good news. I've just finished comparing your last two CAT scans. The lesions are definitely diminishing. Of the six lesions we have been tracking, five have disappeared. No trace of them on these X-rays. All we've got left is this small one here." Both Genie and I held our breath. "We'll keep close watch on it."

Five tumors down and one to go. Genie and I had come a long way. And thanks to the residual effect of IL-2, we still had hope that the remaining tumor would disappear. We needed the amps our "power pack" of Buffaloes could provide to zap this last ornery critter.

September 7, 1990

YO, TEAM BUFFALO!

LATEST SCORE
BUFFALOES - 99.50 CANCER - 00.50

I heard from my doctor yesterday who had just compared my last two CAT scans, measuring how much the lesions on my lungs had diminished. Guess what, Gang? Of the six lesions that we have been tracking five are completely gone!

We go back to Duke on September 30th to begin Game Three. Your support has made the difference so please keep up your thoughts and prayers for this next offensive push.

I think about the Real Red bike a great deal, and when OUR TEAM wins it, you can ride it anytime —squirrel tail handlebars and all!

Thanks again!

Love, Bob

And out in the territory where the Buffaloes roamed, squirrel tail mania broke out.

The tails for the handlebars of our Real Red bike were proving to be a major headache for our Chief Scribe. Jenny set up camp on her back deck in Atlanta, hoping to entice a squirrel into surrendering its anterior. But the squirrels got wise that Jenny was on their tail. The branches of the trees stilled as the high flyers elected to stay put. The grape arbor which provided a nocturnal playground for the wildlife in the deeply suburban neighborhood suddenly became as deserted as an old Lucy and Desi set.

The boycott left Jenny with only one choice. Forget the promised squirrel tails, Jenny decided. The leaves were off the trees now and a winter chill tightened its grip. In desperation, Jenny enlarged her sweep for handlebar accessories. She went after raccoons.

Jenny was driving past a strip shopping center when she spotted Eddie's Trick Shop. Jenny braked and bolted inside. Boy, it was sure going to take a neat trick to pull off what she was after. "Do you have any squirrel tails?" Jenny asked, hopefully.

Eddie's bulbous fake nose lit up like a Vegas slot machine. "Nope, all out."

"How about raccoon tails? Jenny pressed on doggedly. "I need something for the handlebars of a bike."

Eddie brightened. He was following right along with her train of thought, Jenny could see. A stream of water spurted from an enormous flower in Eddie's lapel. His nose went to neon again, and from somewhere in his great, generous chest, a Woody Woodpecker laughed crazily. "You're in luck! I've got raccoon caps!"

"You mean like Davy Crockett wore?" Jenny asked.

"Why not? You can cut the tails off the caps!" Eddie said, triumphantly. Maniacal laughter erupted. Eddie grabbed for his shears.

Thanks to the trappers of Cherokee, North Carolina and Eddie, Jenny soon had a pair of jaunty raccoon tails. She also had two Davy Crockett caps *sans* tails which were recycled as Russian fur hats for the winter ahead.

The Stones had a lot to be thankful for. And did we evermore know it!

November 22, 1990

Dear Team,

Happy Thanksgiving! The Stones have a great deal to be thankful for this year, and you are at the top of the list. Nine months ago when I asked you to take this journey with me, I had no idea that we would come from a score of Buffaloes 25 - Cancer 75 to our present tally of Buffaloes 99.5 - Cancer 00.50. This has been accomplished by the best medical care and knowledge and care available, an incredibly strong and supportive family, your thoughts and prayers, and a loving God who has answered them. I am one thankful guy to have family and friends like you.

Going For the Win

Yogi Berra best summed up my last treatment at Duke when he said, "It was like deja vu all over again." I won't bother you with my "war story" but will simply say that my ole body could only take 11 of the 15 days of IL-2 treatment. We had hoped to get rid of the last remaining lesion on my right lung, but the CAT scan I had last week showed that it was still there. The good news is that it did not grow—we will continue to watch it on a monthly basis. In the meantime, Genie has me on a rigorous exercise program and a very nutritious diet. I feel good and my strength is coming back daily. We are extremely optimistic about the future.

Word from my cousin Jenny is that I am still in contention for the REAL RED bike which is still my main goal. With your continued support we'll win it!

The enclosed picture of the home team was made on our trip this summer out West. When you look at it know that Genie, Tyler, Marion and I love you and wish for you a very Merry Christmas and a joyous 1991!

Love, Bob

TWELVE

A Boy's Christmas

This is the story of a boy's Christmas. Christmas Day, 1990
was a record breaker on all fronts. Genie had outdone herself
decking the halls. Our farm house was endangered by the sheer
weight of mistletoe, holly, pine boughs, and answered prayers.
The remaining tumor on my lung had disappeared completely. My
cancer was in remission.

Our daughter Marion, who had given up a year of her life to
bear with her parents, was on her way to her new career as a
counselor in an outdoor program for teenagers at-risk. She had
certainly been a key player in her dad's recovery. Tyler came
roaring up the mountain for the holidays, filling every room with
his infectious laughter. Genie was painting again. A portrait of Tyler
was in progress on her easel, unquestionably her best work. And
Santa Claus was coming to town!

We had finished opening the family gifts on Christmas
morning when Tyler suddenly ducked out the front door without
explanation. He returned, pushing the shiniest Real Red bike this
old boy had ever seen! Two luxuriant raccoon tails dangled from
the handlebars. WE HAD WON! This note was attached:

Christmas Day
December 25, 1990

FROM: Tripp Winn with Schwinn Bicycle
Company

CONGRATULATIONS, MR. BOB STONE!

Our own independent audit has verified that you are indeed the winner of The Schwinn Mountain Bike Competition. While we were told to hold MTB # REAL RED for January delivery we have little control over the matter. A Red Bike is like a divining rod. It will find a boy and his Christmas in spite of carelessly thought-out schedules. Every red bike we assemble knows exactly where to go. We have observed this phenomenon time and time again. Mr. Bob, can you just picture it! Our Schwinn MTB # REAL RED, jaunty raccoon tails flying, streaking down the highway, over hill and hollow, dirt roads and gullied paths to find its rightful place with you on this Christmas Day! Ms. Stone-Humphries was right about one thing: the Giverny blue bike would never have made it.

May the joy and peace of this season be with you and yours. The SCHWINN COMPANY and the undersigned sponsors wish you the merriest Christmas ever.

Happy Pedaling,

YOUR TWINS, JENNY HUMPHRIES
and BETTY ROBINSON

YOUR POWER PRAYER WARRIORS
DAVID GRIMES
LARRY SITTON
VIC COCHRAN

THIRTEEN

Expansion Teams

The steps in building a team like the Buffaloes have been in use since our Native American coaches first showed us which end of a lacrosse racket to swing.

> Put out a call for a team. Explain the game. Equip
> the team for play. Give everyone a chance to get
> off the bench and participate.

All we have done is to recycle a tried and true team concept to approach life's big challenges. This only illustrates the versatility of the human species.

Building a team for one of life's challenges enables us to take a fresh look at the people around us and bring them together in a community who share their lives, their prayers, their weaknesses, their humanity. This is what we are put here to do. We simply get so busy that we forget the game plan.

No one has understood our "team" concept more than our good friend, Jean Winje (remember the special issue Buffalo postcard she claimed for the team?). Jean and her husband, Larry, are members of our couples study group within our Northwestern family. No one should have to go it alone, Jean believes. Jean gracefully expresses what we have tried to do and what we hope to do in encouraging others to move out, be fruitful and multiply.

Dear Bob,

I've composed letters in my heart to you so many times over the past weeks. It's time to put pen to paper.

I loved your first letter giving "homework" assignments. Well, shoot, Bob, I didn't know at age 45 I'd appreciate "homework." That in itself makes you extra special--the fact that I'm enjoying the assignment must be because the mentor (Bob Stone) has a much more positive approach to life than my other teachers. Must have something to do with the difference between a mentor and teacher!

I've been particularly inspired by Siegel's tapes/meditations/writing. Thank you for introducing me to him. Our lives are changing, too, as we become less focused on immediacy and more focused on the broader picture of life. Life itself becomes the gift, and living with the joys and sorrow of friends and family is what it's all about.

I have been repeatedly struck with the beautiful way you have reached out—to invite all of us to participate in your life and the life of your family...

"Study groups" have posed some interesting thoughts for me since becoming a part of the Northwestern Family—what I realize now is that aside from the sharing of business, there is the awesome possibility of sharing intimately with friends, and it is an evolutionary process and it involves commitment and, perhaps, becomes more

precious as we age. The very notion that any one of us has to "do it alone" becomes sillier and sillier the more we are open to the beauty of intimate friendships.

I had this wonderful visual thought about buffaloes and how, try as we did to wipe them out, those dear strong buffaloes are making a forceful comeback! Watch out, Cowboys!!!

By now I hope you, like Jean Winje, are open to the awesome possibility of sharing your life with others, and are sold on the team concept to tackle a hefty challenge in your own life. Perhaps you have formed your own team or become a part of someone else's team. Fun, hope, compassion, inspiration: all these good things are meant to be shared.

Your own team can be as sparse and lean as a Russian chess team with no alternates or it can be as multifarious and beefy as the Pittsburgh Steelers. You choose. Then take the team concept and run with it. Spin off. Think about building the franchise. Think Expansion Teams!

The Buffaloes found the expansion possibilities were endless. We discovered one life challenge opened the way to another challenge and then to another. We found our window of opportunity as wide as the world.

In Milwaukee a Buffalo found the courage to spin off a team for his own crucial life challenge. My friend, David, stood up in an AA meeting and took the first step in putting his life back together.

Dear Bob,

In your Aug. 30th letter you said, "My point is this —I could not have done it without family and friends—the team concept works!" When I reread that line this morning, it occurred to me that I

*really understood what you meant—today—8 or
10 months ago I'm not sure I would have
understood the real meaning. I understand what
you said because only by the grace of God—and
my new family and friends am I able to continue
my recovery one day at a time.*

(Letter from David Franczyk dated September 26, 1990)

Another Buffalo in Greensboro read the Buffalo Letters to a
group and found the warmth and humor of the team letters
sparked a free-ranging discussion on fear of cancer and other life-
threatening and life-changing illnesses. Florence Gatten wrote:

*Your wonderful letter circulated and inspired...
even read it aloud in our small group Sat A.M...
With that, the dam broke! People acknowledged
their fear (of cancer)... your brilliant letter gave
them "tasks", a shopping list, a guide to how to
be of support.*

(Letter from Florence Gatten dated 3-19-90.)

Some of the spin-offs do not have to do with grave illness.
One of our teammates wanted to make the medical community
more sensitive to a patient's needs and humanize rigid protocols.
Bob Rock took to the reading list I'd assigned like a champion
retriever to a pond full of ducks. Following the lead of Norman
Cousins, Bob Rock was ready to raise the sensitivity of the whole
medical profession by teaching a class on psychoneuroimmunology. (How could we forget that word?)

...I've about decided on another project. As an outgrowth on the study of psychoneuro-immunology, Cousins focused on the importance of effective doctor-patient relationship and the medical school attention essential to focus on this. I am going to write the UCLA Med School Dean and ask what the status of this project is. Depending on what he tells me, I think I would like to pick up on this, first in NC and then perhaps nationally. I have had a certain amount of experience with this sort of thing with my job at Johnson & Johnson and it truly intrigues me. If handled properly it can be made into an everybody-wins deal—and my experience with my present problems assure me that here is plenty of room for improvement.

(Letter from Bob and Eileen Rock dated July 13, 1991)

Groups I speak to across the country are spinning off their own team as fast as Frisbees flying on a sunny Saturday afternoon. It is exciting to see what others are doing. Here are some excerpts from letters I have received to show you how easy it is. If you're into modeling, this sampling should generate enough ideas to get you started on your first letter to your own team or, even better—suggest how you might respond to someone who needs to hear from you. And remember, a simple straightforward approach is all it takes to get the job done.

Last October my neighbors took me to meet a man named Bob Stone...He recommends that when the chips are really down, that it's time to gather all your "Buffaloes" together to form a team...so as you might have guessed by now you are on my team roster...

(Excerpt from letter from Patty White dated February 6, 1992)

I met an inspiring man named Bob Stone in November who introduced me to the idea of starting a team for prayer support in my fight against cancer. His team was called the "Buffaloes." Why? Because they are a dying breed, but they are just about to make a comeback. I like the idea of a newsletter to keep you updated so that you can pray intelligently and also offer other forms of support, if you feel that is what you would like to do.

There are a great deal of studies being done about the relationship between a patient's physical and mental health in overcoming serious disease.

My white cells are pretty low. A great way to get white cells up is through humor. That's right. I love Far Side jokes, Herman, Buffo, Calvin & Hobbes. So send those cards and letters, jokes, anything to put a smile on my face.

Let's see what happens!

(Letter from Diane Lee dated January, 1992)

Dear Friends:

I am writing now to enlist your membership on my battle team which we are calling the "Sharks" or alternatively, the "Northern Buffaloes."

In our correspondence [Bob Stone] has generously shared with me all the things he has done to fight the battle. The notion of organizing

95

your friends and loved ones to help wage the battle was his, and Sal and I thought we would borrow it, with his permission of course. His team was named the Buffaloes, which explains our alternate name because someday we may have a softball game between the Southern Buffaloes and the Northern Buffaloes.

Now for the team's first assignment ...

(Letter from Jon and Sally Wisotzkey dated February 15, 1992)

As you know Kay has been battling cancer for the past year... To help us in our fight, we are asking that you please continue to lift us up even further in prayer and to continue to correspond with us in any manner that would promote healing. This may be letters, cards, pictures of your family, encouraging newspaper clippings, humorous stories, or comic strips—anything you feel is uplifting...We are determined to do all that we can to win this battle, and we know there is strength in numbers. We plan to correspond with you on a continual basis so that you will be updated frequently on our progress.

(Letter from Rob & Kay Van Gorden dated March 16, 1992)

Dear Prayer partner,

I am writing on behalf of my entire family to let you know how Ruth is doing and to thank you for your prayers...Ruth has been talking with a man named Bob Stone who was recently on CBS This Morning. *He has a huge group of people praying for him, which his family called "The Buffalo Club." Every time he felt like giving up he'd remember those who were praying for him, knowing that he couldn't let them down. We are calling our group the Army*

(Letter from Mary Hopkins dated June 10, 1991)

As you can see, for some of us, expansion teams were a result of thoughtful planning. Others, like me, found that a team just happens—as suddenly and unpredictably as a summer shower...

They were the first tomatoes from my garden—gorgeous, sun-kissed, deep red. Genie had promised to make bread in honor of the first home-grown tomato sandwiches of the season, but there was Maggie and her new pups, and those mountain laurels to be planted in the shrub border, and a herd of Buffaloes that left only this morning after a weekend with us. No bread.

"Bob, would you mind going to the store for a loaf?" My wife asked with a tired but totally unnecessary apology in her voice that late afternoon.

"Mind?" I answered. This from a woman who is closing in on the world's record for bearing with a husband in sickness and in health. "Be back in 15 minutes."

I was out the back door like a shot. Outside it was starting to rain. Big soft drops plopped against the windshield.

The three women looked damp and forlorn standing by the side of the road. I could see they weren't locals, their shoes weren't sturdy enough for this hill country. The three looked displaced. They waited patiently, with an air of expectancy, as if they knew the next car coming was their lift. I was the next car coming. I checked the rear view just to make sure. I really didn't want to stop. Surely, someone would be along in a moment.

"Don't even slow down, Bob," I instructed myself firmly. The rain was beginning to pour down. I adjusted my rear view mirror so I could keep the three women in sight. Suddenly the darkness seemed to press down on me, the rain wasn't pleasant, it seemed downright uncomfortable.

I took my big foot off the gas, mad at myself. I'd told Genie I'd be back in fifteen minutes. Ruts of guilt and worry trenched my brow. Cancer loves worry and guilt. It grows on worry and guilt— and on chocolate chip cookies. I snapped the car in reverse. With my luck the three stranded women were probably packing chocolate chip cookies in their suitcases.

"Why are you ladies standing out in the rain?" I asked pleasantly, sticking my head out the car window.

"We're looking for a lift to the bus station." The older woman seemed eager to speak. Her voice was educated, well-modulated and Deep South. The two younger women didn't speak. They simply yanked the door open and crowded into the back seat.

"We've been thrown out," the youngest said sorrowfully.

"Thrown out?"

"From _____." The second one added.

I recognized the name of the recovery facility up the road.

"They were right to throw us out."

"They have their rules."

"We broke the rules. No getting around that."

I listened to this Greek chorus of woe. "What did they nail you for?" I prodded.

"Fraternizing with the guys. They're in another dorm just across the road."

Wouldn't you know it? I thought to myself. They always are.

"What has us worried sick is the timing of this thing. Do you think we've been in the program long enough to do any good?

We've only had about four weeks. We're not too sure we can make it on our own."

"It's a six-week program." The youngest of the three in the back seat chimed in, dejectedly. "We're on our own now. Up the creek without a paddle."

My thoughts reeled back to NCI and those two kids all alone. What had I asked them—*where are your people?* I turned around to look at my wet and bedraggled passengers. Where were their people? What I saw rocked me. I saw the very thing I'd seen one afternoon a year ago in my kitchen with a counter loaded with casseroles. I saw a team already in place. I saw a *team* in the back seat of my car!

"You've already got everything you need to win your fight," I began. You already have a team to see you through. The three of you ARE a team!" I could feel a missionary zeal building inside me. These three could do it. They were strong, recognized the problem, wanted to get on with the program.

I careened past the Quick Stop, heading hellbent for leather to the bus station in town. On the way, I gave them my full presentation on team building.

I felt my stomach lurch as I pulled into our driveway more than an hour later. Guiltily, I glanced at my watch and hurried inside. Chin in hand, my wife was staring at those first homegrown tomatoes on the kitchen table, as if waiting for them to speak. "Where's the bread?" she looked at me glumly.

I was out the back door like a shot.

It was weeks later when we were sinking under the weight of those same garden tomatoes that Genie brought in the day's mail. I didn't recognize the handwriting, but when I saw the south Georgia postmark I remembered the spokeswoman for our newest expansion team and her charming Deep South accent. She had taken the team concept to heart. She had gone home, enlisted the members of a local church to be on her team, was continuing her recovery. She wrote that her husband was attending church with her for the first time. Her two companions were doing equally as well.

And Genie willingly forgave all of us!

FOURTEEN

Cancer Is Not the Death Knell

"**S**o what have you learned this past year, Bob. What one thing would you like viewers to know?" CBS producer, Michael Radutzky asked from behind his camera in the *CBS This Morning* interview.

"People need to know that cancer is not a death knell," I began, my hand seeking out Genie's hand. "It can be beaten and here are some of the things I've found to be helpful. You need to get yourself a team."

The hills were alive with the sound of "Roll 'em!" and "That's a wrap!" Fellow Buffalo and televison producer Michael Radusky had brought down his crew with *CBS This Morning* to film one segment of a week-long series Dr. Bob Arnot was doing on cancer. Michael believed our team concept was unique and could benefit others. Both Michael and Bob Arnot wanted viewers across the country to see the team concept in action.

A huge picture board of zany Buffaloes was propped on an easel. The crew had taken a break. Michael and Genie were talking nutrition, Michael's new baby, and homemade apple pie. Michael was into all of it. Things were rocking around the clock!

Genie and I found Dr. Bob Arnot just as knowledgable and genuine sitting across the dinner table as he was on camera. We three guys took to the trails—me on my Real Red MTB with raccoon tails flying straight out at attention and Bob and Michael on loaners.

Dr. Bob Arnot in this special series gave us an in-depth perspective on this pandemic of cancer:

Too many of us are not receiving state-of-the-art care for our cancer. We opt instead for the hometown doctor we play tennis with or meet at church, and the hospital close to home. We are slow to ask questions about treatment or to ask for a second opinion.

Too many of us are failing to do our homework. We refuse to research the hospitals and cancer centers engaged in trials for promising new drugs and experimental treatments. Don't all doctors and hospitals have access to the latest drugs and research? Not always. There are one hundred cancer centers in the US. And about twenty-eight of them are *comprehensive* cancer centers which means these cancer centers are linked directly with the National Cancer Institute and work hand in hand with NCI.

The chances are that your local surburban hospital, however convenient and comfortable it may be, probably is NOT involved in this kind of state-of-the-art treatment. Across the country you will find the trials follow the grant money and grant money follows the doctors involved in research for a particular kind of cancer. These doctors are scattered all across the country in various comprehensive cancer centers and teaching and research hospitals. For example, the Duke Comprehensive Cancer Center is on the cusp of innovative treatment for ovarian cancer. A teaching hospital in Alabama may be doing the latest bone marrow transplants. Of course, you have to fit the protocol—it's chancey, but then, so is cancer.

Too many of us don't know the National Cancer Institute mans a cancer hotline twenty-four hours a day around the clock. USE IT. NCI can advise you of the latest treatment for your cancer, tell you what hospitals are conducting new trials. This information is yours, free of charge, by dialing 1-800 4-CANCER.

WHERE THE BUFFALOES ROAM

Too many of us don't practice basic self defense when it comes to fending off cancer, the CBS report warned us. We smoke, carry too much excess weight. We talk a good game of cholesterol but scarf it up at every opportunity. We drag our feet in scheduling regular physical exams, ignore our family history and genetic disposition toward disease. We can do a lot to improve our odds against cancer by becoming a defensive player.

Too many of us fail to let our congressmen know that we consider cancer appropriations to be of the same priority as a Stealth bomber or pull-down maps for the war room at the Pentagon.

Genie and I made some lasting friendships among the *CBS This Morning* crew and we are proud to have them on our team.

As a result of the *CBS This Morning* interview our telephone went on Ready alert. The series on cancer touched a nerve in those who were fighting or helping someone else fight cancer. Responses and requests for help flooded in.

The staff at the Duke Comprehensive Cancer Center asked me to speak to a Congressional committee on funding for cancer research. I told our North Carolina congressmen they were looking at the best reason I could think of to fund cancer research. "Without research money I would be a memory today," I said.

Groups of cancer survivors, cardiac patients, those with AIDS, and others facing big life challenges have taken me into their hearts and asked me to speak to and *for* them. Some are shy, some are lonely, some are alone. "I could never get a team together," they tell me. My answer is unvarying. You already have a team, I tell them. Look around you. Your team is there. Who did you eat lunch with? Who's on your softball team? Who sits in the pew with you when you worship? Who signed your birthday card at the office? Your team is in place. All it requires is a little organization. Then I see something flare in their eyes that wasn't there before. Hope is contagious and it can metastasize faster than cancer cells.

Most of those I talk with have accepted the diagnosis they have been given. They do not deny it. But what they want is less doom and gloom and a positive stance from the doctors who are treating them. Bernie Siegel, whom I have never met face-to-face, gave me a generous-hearted endorsement when he told Bob Arnot and his television viewers that I had found what so many people were looking for—how to find joy in this moment. This is what all of us fighting a dismal prognosis want—joy in the moment. Because for many, joy—their very life—is measured in that moment.

Weeks later a television crew from Whittle Communications barreled over the mountain pass to film a program on the role of humor in healing, a subject Norman Cousins dealt with in his book, *Anatomy of An Illness*.

And six months after that first *CBS This Morning* interview, Genie and I got another telephone call from CBS producer, Michael Radutzky. "Bob, we were talking about doing something special for Christmas. We asked ourselves, 'Is there one story we have done this year that really stands out?' Bob, you and the Buffaloes were our hands-down choice. Could we come down and do a recap on everyone's favorite story?"

So amid the Christmas festivity of downtown Greensboro the film crew followed us as we shopped at the malls and stopped by First Presbyterian Church where we talked with our pastor, Jerry Shetler. I realized while sitting in that peaceful sanctuary that we had found this very thing through our faith—sanctuary. Our God had not only offered us steadfast refuge, but a way to reach out to others. He had taught us that bad could be turned into positive force to help others. It is one thing to read this in the ancient scriptures but quite another to see it translated into your life.

They even asked Genie what she wanted for Christmas. Her eyes filled with tears. "I've already gotten what I wanted," she said quietly.

And I got what I wanted the day Genie Stallworth said "yes" to a brash young kid fresh out of Davidson College.

FIFTEEN

Another Season

Living life *with* cancer proved to be another season and I was a rookie all over again. My team had helped me through my long ordeal, they coached me, encouraged me, and had given me a swift kick when I needed it. Now we were into a sudden death play-off (not a bad analogy!). In the course of one year we got bonded—and branded—for life. And we weren't done with each other yet.

March 1, 1991

Dear Team:

1990 was the year of the Buffalo! The herd had a starring role in Dances With Wolves; the Buffalo Bills missed winning the Super Bowl by 3 feet; and our TEAM—THE BUFFALOES came on strong in December and won the REAL RED bike in a dramatic finish! Imagine my surprise on Christmas morning when I received the enclosed letter from Jenny, followed by Marion and Tyler wheeling in my new red Schwinn. It was wonderful!

Another Season

When I wrote my first letter to you on March 16, 1990, I had cancer in my left kidney, my lymph glands, my spleen, my liver, and both of my lungs. The strange thing was that I looked good and felt great for an ole dude just six weeks over fifty. Today, I am just six weeks over fifty-one, look good, feel great, and am tumor free! My last scans were very positive. They show only one small shadow on one lung—we can't tell if it's scar tissue or the remains of a shrinking tumor. How did this happen?

In my first letter I mentioned that my parents, my grandparents, and my Sunday School teachers taught me long ago that God is Love, and that I was feeling this love in abundance through your calls, letters, beautiful flowers and positive thoughts. I am here today because of the love I received from you, my family, and the wonderful folks at Duke. Our bumper sticker reads BUFFALOES - UNDEFEATABLE CHAMPS. *We are a powerful team, and I thank GOD every day for you.*

Norman Cousin's book, Head First: The Biology of Hope, *presents the rapidly mounting scientific evidence that hope, faith, love, will to live, purpose, laughter, and festivity can help combat serious illness. Most importantly, such attitudes can enhance the environment of medical treatment. Each of you has helped me with these attitudes. You are my heroes.*

As I did with my first letter, I am again asking the TEAM to do the following things:

1. Please read the following verses from the Bible that have meant so much to me:

Psalms 23:4	*Jeremiah 30:17*
John 6:47	*Psalms 31:24*
Proverbs 8:17	*John 3:16*
Isaiah 55:12	*I John 4:19*
Hebrews 11:1	*John 13:34,35*

2. Please read Head First: The Biology of Hope *by Norman Cousins and give a copy to someone in the medical community or to a friend who has been diagnosed with a serious illness.*

3. Call me if you or anyone you know gets cancer, and you think that I can help. I have met many brave and courageous people this year who have cancer and have given me hope. It is my desire to help anyone at any time. Give me a call.

4. If you haven't already, please send me your picture for the OFFICIAL TEAM PROGRAM. It represents the most powerful team on Earth.

5. My friends at the Duke Cancer Center would love your extra Girl Scout cookies. Send me your extra tickets to the Eastern Regionals!

6. Lastly, but most importantly, remember us in your prayers. You will always be in ours. Genie, Tyler, Marion and I love you very much.

Bob,
Matthew 7:7,8

Another Season

With my cancer in remission, Genie and I were now a part of a larger kingdom—that kingdom of survivors—those who were not dying of cancer but living with cancer. The rights of surviorship are hard to come by and, sometimes, hard to live with.

Many of us survive the toughest fight of our life only to discover that survival can mean the loss of a job, a business, the means of support and self-esteem that we need now more than ever before. For many, it means cancelled or restricted insurance coverage. There is something about cancer and a company's insurance and benefits program that too often spell disaster. Those who have been most supportive when we were dying become distressingly remote when we are back at our desk and the cost of disease must be dealt with long term.

How long I can remain tumor free is anyone's guess. I know the odds. Renal cell carcinoma has a way of showing up again—uninvited and unwelcome, like a cat that won't stay put out. When and if it does come back we'll fight it again.

However, the long-term results and continued survival of those of us who participated in the IL-2 trials are a definite encouragement. I have hope. And a team to see me through whatever comes.

I've thought a lot about why people got caught up in the Buffaloes. I look into the mirror and see a severely middle-aged fellow who's seen the road to enviable good health turn to ruts. Who is this fellow—the rainmaker? Super Motivator? Oozing charisma all over the place, huh?

Nope. I'm an ordinary human being, just like you.

I believe the Buffaloes are proof that we all want to be connected, want to live and work and love something outside of ourselves. Scott Peck, Bernie Siegel, Norman Cousins and others like them have put their finger right on the pulse of this need in our human condition, this dark bituminous vein of yearning. Over the course of my ordeal, what could have been strictly a solo act became a congregational sing-in. One guy became every guy. We all wanted the red bike, we all wanted to reach beyond ourselves and the terminal day-to-day of our lives. We all *hoped* for the same things. And miraculously we found it—in one another.

Suzanne Lewis said it: "I think most people are honored that you care enough about them to let them know what is happening in your life, and most of all that you value their help." How often we are asked for our money, our skills, our contacts, our know-how. How refreshing it is when all someone wants is just *me*. It *is* a privilege to join and share and make ourselves a part of that larger community.

Winning, if it is simply living or dying, is not the criteria. It is that vital sense of being a part of that larger community that renews and allows us to see all of life in a fresh perspective. Bearing with another human being in facing their challenge is what is important.

My team certainly answered the challenge. What was so great about the Buffaloes was that we were able to get back to that essential *me* in each of us. We were like a group of fighter pilots stationed on a remote desert airfield. Money, prestige, position, power—none of that did us any good where we were. What we got back to were the basics, the guy who could tell a good story, the guy who could pitch a game of horseshoes, or play a game of cards or make you laugh, or cry, or think. How rare it is that we are ever asked to be that quintessential *me* with another person. And that's exactly what I asked for when I asked others to join my team. Let's get reacquainted with that pal I hit it off with in college, that guy who first showed me my best lay up shot, the kid who split his popcorn and malt balls with his dad at the movie show. What I wanted from each person on my team was the *kindredness* that attracted us in the first place. I wanted the friend they wanted to be.

Of course, many of those I first met while building my team were people who were like me. They had cancer. I camped out with them on the Jordan Ward at Duke, and we campaigned together during long weeks of therapy. I have visited with them in their homes. But what amazes me is the way everyone caught hold of that larger vision of the Buffaloes and carried it out into their everyday affairs. The trickle-down effect.

Experiencing life first hand is invigorating. Joining with others is energizing. Albert Schweitzer wrote:

> *In helpfulness to others, every man can find, on his own doorstep, adventure for the soul—our surest source of peace and lifelong satisfaction.*

Ever talk with a guy who has crewed one of the boats in the America's Cup challenge? He is running out the seams with strategy, ploys, go-for-broke stunts. He's so filled with life's *answered* challenge that it's strictly a judgement call whether he won or lost. He played in the game, he experienced it! It is this *answer* to a challenge that builds our sense of worth and self-esteem and makes life worthwhile for as long as we have it.

I've discovered that at the core, people are lonely. If we aren't talking the same God, you may attribute this loneliness to man's alienation from his society, a highly technological society that is at a far remove from the most basic needs of the human heart.

If we are talking the same God, you have a theology to match this condition. The condition is the separation of man from God. We have been left with a God-sized hole in our heart. But we can do a lot of back-filling when we allow ourselves to love others the way God loves us. Hard, unconditionally, and for life.

And one of the ways I have found to cure that alienation that is within all of us is by being a friend and asking someone else to be your friend. You have to be a friend to make a friend. We all learned that in grade school. I relearned it with this audacious, bodacious, intrepid herd of Buffaloes who wouldn't accept extinction and didn't much like interlopers like cancer in their territory.

SIXTEEN

The Underground Movement

The most remarkable of all that has come out of that extraordinary year with the Buffaloes is the underground movement circulating the Buffalo letters. These letters have come to have a life of their own.

One person reads the letters, thinks of a friend who is going through a life-changing ordeal. He in turn passes the letters along to his friend as a way of nurturing hope. The letters are a testament of one passing, ongoing from rivulet to stream and on and on, until finally we glimpse the great headwaters—and what are the great headwaters? Our humanity. A mighty force that has as its source the single individual has now formed and reformed us irrevocably into that larger body. The force of our combined humanity is awesome.

And what is it that has so moved us to join together—is it mere affliction? No, I don't think so. It is not even the passage of Life to Death. It is the *passing* itself; the stately, clumsy, heartbreaking, joyous passing through this life. And we cannot make it without Hope. We cannot make it without one another. And I believe this is how one man becomes Every Man—in the marking and sharing of that passing.

I believe the Buffalo letters caught on for a simple reason. Big medicine too often extinguishes the very thing it tries to sustain. Life, hope, the will to go on. I do not mean to denigrate medicine. I owe my life to big medicine and to those who practice it.

But medicine as we have it today is merely a reflection of the world around us. Population has exploded, cities have grown, specialization and technology have mushroomed. Our world is very specialized, our skills are also. And this specialization has separated us from the whole. In short, all of us have suffered a loss of community, and that includes those who practice medicine. Medicine has been broken down into innumerable state-of-the-art specialties practiced by doctors with extremely defined skills. It takes some doing to retrieve the whole person, for both doctor and patient. But it can be done.

Somewhere out there is someone who has been diagnosed with cancer. He slumps in a chair at home in front of the TV; depressed, unable to eat, totally without the will go on. Why should he, when he has been told he will not go on? He has lost that essential feeling that he still has control of his life. Somehow his life no longer belongs to him. His life is loaded on a gurney, examined by specialists, monitored, sealed in the capsule of a huge impersonal CT scanner. Where is the ME in all of this, he wonders.

I wish for him that same kind of support I've had from my team. Here is a man who isn't afraid to die; he simply has no will to become so much medical chattel. He wants dignity. He needs to know that he can still choose. He can choose how he wants to face his mortality, who he wants to face it with. The choice is his, just as surely as he can choose what kind of grass to sow on his lawn. And once he discovers he *can* choose, he begins to eat, puts on a little weight. He feels better physically, he begins to see friends, leave his chair and television. He reclaims himself from the wreckage of this terminal accident which had his name on it.

It is this loss of person which incapacitates us and renders us incapable of going on.

I have a ninetysomething year old Uncle Charlie who is very dear to me. Recently he was hospitalized, had surgery, rallied, then inexplicably grew weaker in the hospital day by day. It was his housekeeper who put her finger on his downhill slippage. "They don't allow him his dignity," she said. "A gentlemen like your uncle needs his own pajamas, his robe, his slippers, his *things—*

you know what I'm talking about?"

I certainly did. And back home in his own pajamas, his robe and his slippers, my uncle made rapid recovery.

My cousin Jenny has a very courageous friend who has lived with cancer for almost thirty years. Betty has battled the disease into remission so many times that she must feel like a heroine in a televison soap opera. Even when her cancer is aggressively active, she continues on, as she is able. She sees her friends. She attends vocational courses at her community college, she does freelance work at home on her computer. She continues. She hopes. One feeds the other in perfect symbiotic balance. And that balance is crucial in a long-term confrontation.

SEVENTEEN

Coming Around Again

When a matador survives his afternoon of blood and sand, he is awarded the ears and tail of the freight train on hoof that tried to run him down. I got something even better.

The parcel UPS delivered was as large and bulky as the Bunyan-sized duffle bag I had hauled over to Germany as a GI. And about as heavy. "What on earth!" Genie laughed, as we took a walking tour around it.

"A compact car," I offered.

We cut the string on the box—inside was a mass of dark, dense fur, and the unmistakable scent of the wild. Genie and I unrolled the bundle then stood back, awed.

We were looking at the hide of one enormous buffalo. Let me tell you those fellows are BIG!

Genie put her arm around my shoulders and said, "Buffalo Bob, This one's for you."

I could barely hold back my tears as I gazed at that magnificent hide—what length, what breadth, what stupendous power on the hoof! I leaned over and took another good deep breath of that noble beast. My buffalo.

Now the hide hangs along the stairs leading to a study. It stretches almost the whole length of the staircase. Each time I pass, I dig my fingers into it and find comfort in its rough thickness. It is like an old soul, a friend of mine said.

The members of my team have a non-cancellable ticket good for a ride on the red bike anytime they want. And they take me up on the offer! We get picnickers, bikers, hikers, tag-alongs. Many have dropped by to kick tires on the bike, check out those snazzy raccoon tails, talk about their winning season. The one coming up.

We Buffaloes believe all that goes around comes around. Since our story started with the great Allied General, Field Marshall Ferdinand Foch, it only seems right that the Field Marshall has the last word.

Our situation is excellent. We are attacking.

Letters

Thursday, February 22, 1990

Dear Bob,

You are a hard man to catch up with and I sure understand why. Missed you at both home and office. Then Betty talked with Genie and got an update.

We have really been rocked by what has happened, as I am sure you have been too, in spades. We do not accept this! I am sorry that you are being deluged with phone calls from all of us who feel the same way. This is what you get for leading a good upright life—if you were a scum-bag nobody would care. And we do.

Please know that we are concerned for you and for Genie and the kids. Whether it's Duke or NCI, I feel like you are in a really good place to get the best treatment. And I know that same fellow who sold the most subscriptions and won the bike (in the Kids Campaign) is going to win again.

I leave you with Field Marshal Foch's pithy communication from the front during The Great War:

> *My center is giving way, my right is in retreat. Situation is excellent. I am attacking.*

Guess who won? You better believe it!

Love, Jenny

March 16, 1990

Dear Family and Friends,

I received the letter on the previous page from my cousin one week after getting my major "wake-up call", and I laugh every time I read the last paragraph. It describes very well the attitude of the Stone camp. We are attacking—and each of you is helping us in this battle more than you know.

My parents, my grandparents, and my Sunday School teachers taught me long ago that God is love. Genie, Tyler, Marion and I have felt God's love in abundance through your hugs, your tears, your wonderful letters and cards, your calls, beautiful flowers, delicious food, fantastic chocolate chip cookies, pictures and happy banners for my hospital room, but especially through your prayers. God has shown His love through you—and I love you for it!

Now for a up-to-date report.

Physically - *I feel fantastic and look great for an old dude just six weeks over fifty. We have been hiking four to six miles every day for the last week. I could whip any hot-shot handball player if my doc would let me play. I have no loss of appetite, blood pressure is normal. In short, you would think that this guy is looking good.*

Mentally - *From the moment I knew I had renal cell carcinoma, I went on the attack. There has been no depression, no anger, no fear, just desire to get the gears rolling. With the aid of the caring, fast-moving Greensboro medical community, we had the wheels turning in short order.*

Spiritually - *From the very beginning, I have had a sense of peace. I have prayed for strength and God has delivered that through family, our Pastor, close friends, my staff, and all of you who care. We feel very blessed.*

We've had a slight change of plans. The National Institutes of Health is no longer in the picture. We feel that Duke is the right place for us. I am scheduled to be at Duke next Tuesday, and we're hoping for some quick decisions on my treatment there. We will send you all a postcard to let you know firm plans and an address as soon as we get the word.

The Stones would like for you to help us in our challenge, and I am asking you to do the following things:

1. Please read the following verses from the Bible: Ps. 23:4, John 6:47, Prov. 8:17, Is. 55:12, Heb. 11:1, Jer. 30:17, Ps. 31:24, John 3:16, John 13:34, 35, 1 John 4:19.

2. Please read some or all of the following books: Anatomy of An Illness *and* Head First: The Biology of Hope *by Norman Cousins;* Love, Medicine, and Miracles *and* Peace, Love, and Healing *by Bernie Siegel, MD (also on tape);* Healing Yourself *by Martin Rossman, MD.*

119

3. Be thinking—when I get a hospital address, I would like for you to send me pictures—of you, your children, your grandchildren, your parents, your pets, your current girl or boy friends or friends; cards or letters telling me what you're doing, what's happening with your family, business, school, your career plans, who you think will be in the Final Four, funny stories. Think about making tapes reminding me of fun times we've had together, jokes, and the funniest thing that has ever happened to you (we hold everything in confidence). Draw pictures for my room. I want to smile and laugh a great deal!

4. Please send your leftover Girl Scout cookies. I understand my colleagues and the staff at the Duke Comprehensive Cancer Center have a ferocious appetite!!

5. Please call the weather station and leave us messages. We will have weather updates and I love to hear your voices.

6. Lastly, but most important, remember us in your prayers. You will certainly be in ours.

Love, Bob

Letters

March 21, 1990

Dear Family and Friends,

LET THE GAMES BEGIN!

Q. When do the games begin?
A. March 22, 1990
Q. Where are the Open ceremonies being held?
A. Duke University Cancer Center.
Q. What is the first event?
A. Radical nephrectomy of a wonderful, but tired left kidney.
Q. What is the time of the event?
A. Friday morning, March 23.
Q. Where will the team reside?
A. Our address is:
Q. From a long-time Charlotte/Davidson friend—Will there be writs or review on the Bible verses or books recommended?
A. Your work is pledged.
Q. What kind of jokes shall I send in? Are one-liners okay?
A. Sure. It's better to have loved a short girl than never love a tall.
Q. From a homely-looking high school buddy—will my baby picture do?
A. Absolutely—I prefer it!
Q. How long will the first event last?
A. The team will be at Duke until March 30.
Q. What is the next venue?
A. Four to six weeks training at the beach and in the mountains.
Q. What next?
A. Back to Duke for the main event. Friendly competition with the protocol.
Q. How long will it last?

A. Two weeks.
Q. What are the side effects?
A. I'll look like the Pillsbury Dough Boy or the Michelin Tire Man for awhile, but I understand the wide look is coming back in.
Q. How do we get an update?
A. Call the weather station.
Q. Do Bob, Genie, Tyler and Marion love you?
A. ABSOLUTELY— and we appreciate your continued support!

Love, Bob

Wednesday, March 21, 1990

Dear Bob,

After your call I realized that we are really messing up big time. We've let you go up against the Duke Medical juggernaut without selecting our marching song, the music we will be known by. Even little David was accompanied by a lyre. Bob, we've got to have an anthem which will identify our Movement. All the good movements have them. "We Shall Overcome" comes readily to mind but it's been done to death.

I believe you will agree that our anthem should sound the ringing Calvinist tones of our faith. What we want is a song that is Presbyterian but also just a little raunchy. I offer my nomination, Keith Whitley's It Ain't Nothing. *You guys who belong to the Pickup and RV crowd may be all over this one but just in case a tape is enclosed. I think it sort of fits a Bob Stone— laid back, an easy rhythm which is of crucial importance in your present situation, if I read you.*

In my earlier letter we talked about winning and prizes. But details were omitted. You have convinced me that you are serious about winning so let's go for the gold. There is really only one prize worth winning.

IT'S A SCHWINN, BOB!

This bike is being offered through a special arrangement with the Schwinn Company, official outfitters of Stone Expeditions for half a century.

The bike is fully loaded and customized to your exact specifications. It is turbo-charged. The

123

brakes have been stripped from this particular model so that upon reaching optimum racing speed there is, quite literally, no stopping you.

It comes with fringed driving gloves and white sidewall sneakers with steel toes (remember no brakes).

Custom trim kit includes two squirrel tails for the handlebars. Pony skin saddle seat for that touch of pure luxury. Aerial for your flag (It goes whoosh, whoosh!). Included as standard equipment are two clothes pins and a pack of Bicycle playing cards which also make snazzy wheel covers. Mud flaps with 2 glo-lite glass studs for inclement weather complete the package.

*Other lesser prizes: Sylvester Stallone's boxing trunks, a lifetime subscription to GRIT, the bestseller,*The Six Week Cholesterol Cure *(the remedy is severe, as you already know first hand), a heavy duty truss (for when things start slipping). We even offer a splendid consolation prize: Eternal Glory (awarded with two (2) Oak Leaf Clusters).*

But Bob the prize you want is the bike. It's red.

Love, Jenny

April 5, 1990

Dear Family and Friends,

There were six bright, pretty, very verbal and extremely humorous granddaughters in the Stone Family when I arrived in 1940. My two sisters and four cousins welcomed me with loving opened arms, because I brought to their creative world of play the one missing ingredient—a male. The summertimes we spent together were full of fun and adventure. I would do anything they wanted me to do with a smile, because the girls convinced me that's what the role of a little brother/cousin should be. I worked a lot. I can remember my mother playing a jazzed-up wedding march on the piano, as I was the preacher, the groom, and ringbearer in one of our many gala weddings! In short, these young laldies were and still are world-class motivators. Jenny's done it again, folks. I WANT THAT RED BIKE!

On March 16, I wrote to you asking to help the Stones with our challenge and listed some things to do. Tody I'm asking you to join the team that now has an organizational structure. Before giving you the specifics let me tell you how the Opening Ceremonies turned out.

The Duke University Medical Staff showed up in its finest regalia and performed a world-class radical nephrectomy in record time (3 1/2 hours, I am told). The nursing staff was the best! Their professional ability along with a loving, caring manner helped me and my family get through some rough waters. The atmosphere at Duke is perfect for healing.

125

My room did not look like a hospital room at all except for some fellow in the bed hooked up to a lot of hoses. Your drawings, cards, flowers, banners, and especially the photographs made my room the brightest in all of Duke Hosptial. Some friends from Hickory sent a 3'x4' map of the USA entitled "Stone Camp—People, Places, and Prayers." We put flags where all you folks live. My room was a happy place to visit and I thank you for it!

Now for the specific data on OUR TEAM.

The General Manager and Team Physician—The Lord God

As General Manager, He has been impressed with our showing in the first event. As the Team Physician, His fee is small, but His work is priceless.

Head Coach—Genie Stone

Assistant Head Coaches—Tyler and Marion Stone

Team Name—The Buffaloes

Tough ole dudes with a will to live, as evidenced by their remarkable comeback over the last 100 years.

Genie, Tyler, Marion and I thank you for your continued loving support.

Love, Bob
I Corinthians 13:13

126

Letters

April 23, 1990

Dear Team,
          LET THE GAMES CONTINUE!
Q. When do they begin?
*A. As you read this, our team, the Buffaloes, is
on the offensive and attacking the cancer with the
best gameplan known for kidney cancer: Inter-
leukin-2 plus LAK cells.*
Q.What is the current score?
A. The Buffaloes - 97   Cancer - 3
*The surgery on March 23rd removed 97% of the
cancer which was located in the left kidney and
several lymph nodes. We need to work on the
remaining 3% so that the Final Score will be: The
Buffaloes - 100   Cancer - 0.*
Q. How do we win?
A. In short, a TEAM effort
          1. Faith in God
          2. Faith in our medical team and IL-2
          3. Positive attitudes
          4. Prayer
Q.   How can we learn more about IL-2?
A. The May issue of Ladies Home Journal *has an
article, "Lee Remick's Quiet Fight," which
describes exactly what IL-2 is and the recovery
process. Ms. Remick, like the Stones, is fortunate
to have had strong support from family and
friends. It is a good article.*
Q. Isn't the plural of Buffalo Bison?
*A. Yes. But Go-o-o-o Buffaloes sounds better
than Go-o-o-Bison!*
Q. Have the Stones been smiling and laughing?
*A. Absolutely! Your cards, letters, photos,
tapes, videos, cartoons of The Far Side, Calvin
and Hobbes, Cathy, numerous jokes,* You're a
Redneck If, Anguished English, *and other books*

have kept us laughing. I have them all with me now and will need them over the next two weeks!

Q. Did Craig Shergold break the Guinness Book of World Records?

A. Yes. With the help of most of you team members, Craig shattered the old record of 1,265,000 with over 5,000,000 cards, as of April 20. The Children's Wish Foundation expects that he will eventually receive over seven million cards. Thanks for helping.

Q. Should we look over our reading list again?

A. Yes. Reading the scripture verses again and again has helped me. Also, Head First, the Biology of Hope *by Norman Cousins is excellent, and you will be glad you read it.*

Q. Are you charging to see the scar?

A. Yes. $1.00 to the public--FREE to Team Members!

Q. What is my wish?

A. My wish is that I could thank each one of you personally for what you have meant to me, Genie, Tyler, and Marion over the last two months. God has shown us His love through each of you--It has been a wonderful experience. It is my hope that in the future we may be able to return God's love to you, a loved one, or a friend, if a life-threatening disease is experienced. We have learned that you cannot deny the diagnosis, but with faith in God, medical technology and the will to live, you can defy the outcome.

Q. Where does the Red Mountain Bike come in?

A. When I win the bike, you can ride it anytime. It's a fine bike!

Love, Bob
Romans 8:37-39

Letters

May 9, 1990

Dear Bob,

You have been real sick. Everybody says. We are so sorry and would do anything to help you if we could, but this seems to be very much like Lindbergh's flight over the Atlantic—all alone with barely enough light to read his maps, not much food, and not feeling too great. But Lord!—that moment when he saw the sun shining off the coast of France and realized that he'd made it!

My friend wanted me to go with her to see the movie, Glory. I told her to save her popcorn, that it was being enacted in awful living color with real live heroes in Duke hospital even as we spoke. Bob Stone carries our regiment flag, I said, and we don't look for it to fall, or touch ground. It IS hanging pretty low but that is on account of the rough terrain and hazardous footing. But the boy is brave and has good shoes. I am plenty worried, but you can keep your white hanky in your breast pocket, I said to her.

Bob, do you remember when all the Stone Boys had to special order their shoes (Size 15 up) from Winston-Salem and the clerk would call long distance to Stoneville with the message: TELL THE STONE BOYS THEIR SHOES ARE HERE. Well, I think you got your shoes out of the same lot as the rest of those big, gallant men we so loved. Yes, Bob Stone your shoes are here and they aren't easy to fill. Know it.

Tom Robinson talked to one of his doctor friends the other day and he said, if he can stand the treatment, live through this, he's got it licked. Amen.

I am in constant contact with the Schwinn people. We have another contender who broke out of the pack like a Buffalo. He looked real good briefly, then faded. The red bike was an eye-catcher but it turned out he didn't believe in anything—not red bikes, not God, not nothing. He got cured of his cancer but lost the whole point of the game. He didn't think there was a point or really much of a game. Well you better believe that our outfitters at Schwinn think there is a point. That's why they advertise in BOYS LIFE. So it looks like the Buffaloes are trampling all competition by simply being mulish which they have learned from hanging out and being sociable.

Anyway, the Schwinn people wanted to know if we wanted red metallic paint on the bike—flame, they called it. I told them we wanted it to be REAL RED and they are working on it. Thus far the score is in your favor. You have the most points earned and there's no doubt about it. I can almost feel that pedal power under foot. Can you?

Bob I want so badly to help you. I sat down last night and thought what would I want if I were up against it. And like magic I was seven years old and sitting on a creek bank, feeling cool moss like velvet under my bare feet. I was a strong and mighty brave, I could see in the dark, I wasn't afraid. Because in my hand I had a secret weapon. Only me and God knew about it. I pass it along to you.

Enclosed is what every stalwart Prayer Warrior needs: a shotgun shell loaded with Scripture. Not just any Scripture but the verses you have particularly asked us to read. Every verse is packed in this shell and ready to be fired. I put it on a rawhide thong taken from the hide of one mean buffalo. The mere sight of this super-charged shell around your neck is enough to make those C-Cells run. This is heavy duty power. This is magic. This is the power of Our Lord in a magnum shell.

Keep campaigning hard. Go with God and give 'em hell, Bob.

Love, Jenny

WHERE THE BUFFALOES ROAM

May 17, 1990

Dear Team,

There is no place like home! Having spent the last three and a half weeks in the hospital, you can imagine what it is like to get to your own bed, eat home-cooked food and smell fresh air. It's wonderful!

First let me thank you again for your cards, letters, jokes, pictures, and prayers that you sent to pull the team through. We made it, Gang, with flying colors, but with some difficulty at the end. Jenny's letter referred to me as a sick man. This was because I had to go to intensive care for three days at the end of my IL-2 treatment. I was in la-la land—some funny stores to tell here. At any rate, we are now ready to get back in shape for the next round.

Secondly, you need to know that Genie, Tyler, and Marion did an outstanding job of coaching. You team members were terrific support. I am a lucky man!

Q. When will you know if IL-2 Plus LAK did the job?
A. We'll have answers sometime in June.
Q. What will be the next step?
A. Not sure, but will drop you a postcard when certain.
Q. What is the South Carolina state fossil?
A. Strom Thurmond - courtesy of Charlotte Observer.
Q. Is it mandatory to use the Buffalo bumper sticker?

132

A. No. Avid team member from VA printed 500 with the following suggestions:

    1. Use as bumper sticker to invite discussion on how one family is fighting cancer.

    2. Keep for your next scavenger hunt.

    3. Perfect for 1990 time capsule.

Q. What is the best medicine I've had?

A. Laughter is the best medicine.

We will be renewing our physical strength and renewing our spiritual strength in the mountains, but wish you all a lovely spring, happy graduations, wonderful weddings, and much joy, love, and peace.

Love, Bob
Romans 8:28

June 16, 1990
Dear Team,
        LET THE GAMES CONTINUE!
                Score
        THE BUFFALOES 98   CANCER 2
The word from our doctor at Duke is "That we're
on the right track." We were very happy to get
this news and to learn that the IL-2 Plus LAK cell
treatment has caused the tumor on my lung to
shrink. We go back for tests on July 2, 3, and 9.
On July 16th, the Team suits up again for our
second offensive push which will end August 3.
Genie, Tyler, Marion and I are very grateful to
you for your efforts to date, and ask that you
stay in training and gear up for this next push.
Your support means SO much.

To say that we are enjoying the mountains would
be an understatement. Genie has had a wonderful
time in her flower garden and has had a little
time for her painting. Marion has a part-time job
in Blowing Rock and has been doing a great deal
of hiking with our new ten month old puppy,
Maggie. Tyler continues to work for
Northwestern Mutual Life in Charlotte and joins
us on the weekends. I continue to gain my
strength and enjoy Genie's cooking. We are all
excited about a family fishing trip to Montana the
last week in June. Look out trout!

I hope that your spring has been a good one and
that your Summer plans are taking shape. We
have enjoyed hearing from you and being brought
up-to-date on the news from you and your
families. You are good friends.

134

A bit of British humor:
Johnny (to his mother): "I don't want to go to school today.
Mother: "Why not? You haven't been for five days."
Johnny: "The girls tease me, the boys bully me, the staff are unsympathetic."
Mother: "Pull your socks up, Johnny, you're 49 now and the headmaster."

Word from my cousin Jenny is that the Buffaloes are still trampling the competition, and things continue to look good for winning the red Schwinn bike! I'm wearing my secret weapon she sent and campaigning hard. Your continued support and prayers mean MORE than you know. We continue to feel very blessed.

Love, Bob
Exodus 23:25

P.S. Norman Cousin's book, Head First, The Biology of Hope *is on the best seller list. Read it and give it to a friend.*

WHERE THE BUFFALOES ROAM

July 11, 1990

Dear Bob,

I know you are getting ready for another big push in the games. Word is that the bumper stickers are going like hot cakes in Africa. Stan is hot and hungry and speaking French like a pro. We are all preparing to suit up in case you need us to come off the bench and throw a few key blocks for you. While you were off fishing I've had my trials down here. Tripp Winn from the Schwinn Company called the other day. It went like this:

Ms. Stone-Humphries, Winn with Schwinn here. I've the latest communication from our Bob Stone in hand. What a pip of a fight! We've all been following it. You can be sure all of us here are readying for another massive push *to get Bob Stone through his ordeal and back to—wherever. I believe he topped his own personal best in this last round of the games. I thought we'd lost him right at the last. He's recovering at home?*

Nope, Montana. Where the you-know-what roam and seldom is heard a discouraging word.

To be Sure. I must say our man, Bob Stone is not easy to keep track of. It certainly hasn't been easy to keep on top of his progress toward Total Wellness. You spoke of his flying all alone over the Atlantic, of magnum shotgun shells and Indian warriors, carrying the regimental colors into the face of unbelievable odds—the boy has

136

good shoes? Gracious, even the outfitters of Stone expeditionary forces are awed! Where is Bob Stone we ask daily—in the air, on land or at sea?

Yep. Now about the bike, Have you got the bugs worked out of that Real Red? What's the delay in sending down the latest paint samples?

Let's talk about that Real Red you requested. We really can't spray on the final color until we know exactly who has won the machine. I mean fair is fair. An open competition, right? I mean that's what the Schwinn Company has built its reputation on—a fair race among fair-minded boys. We like to think of all of our boys as being physically strong, mentally fit, morally straight— in a word, Ms. Stone-Humphries, all our boys have good shoes!

Tripp, don't make me go over to a competitor. I saw a nifty mountain bike in the L.L. Bean catalog.

You can't be serious! L.L. Bean makes GUM SHOES AND DUFFLES. Schwinn makes cycling machines. I broach the matter of the paint as a simple practicality. What if we go with Real Red and the winner were disappointed? Bob won't be disappointed. It's free. What I'm getting to is simply this. Your Bob Stone may not win the bike. Someone else could come on strong and take it. And what if he or she did not want a Real Red bike. What if their taste ran to a more whimsical color? Our Giverny Blue has been a runaway hit this season.

Tripp, no one whose taste runs to Giverny Blue has a chance of winning your bike. Know it. Besides no one is coming on stronger than our man, Bob.

He could lag in the home stretch—the thought gives me chilblains. He could have equipment failure.

He's already had *equipment failure. Didn't faze him. He blew a tire in the homestretch this last time in Duke. Genie did have to get down off the handlebars but that was the extent of the damage control. Let's see one of your Giverny Blue crowd match that. Besides red is the color we want. Red is the color of courage. As in* Red Badge *of...Red is the Fun Color. Look at fire engines, electric trains, wagons, trikes, sports cars.*

Enough, enough, Ms. Stone-Humphries. I'm weary of the debate. I'll give the shop the go-ahead on Real Red.

Good. Now we can go on to the next thing on the list.

What's that?

Squirrel tails.

Squirrel tails?

For the handlebars. What kind of winter are they predicting up there, Tripp? We like em bushy.

KEEP YOUR EYE ON THE PRIZE, BOB STONE!!!
Love, Jenny

138

August 30, 1990

Dear Team,

I hope this letter finds you in good health with many happy and interesting memories from your summer experience. We have heard about the wonderful weddings, trips to camp, the beach, the mountains, and the fishing outings. Our trip to Montana could not have been more fun, and it looks as though Tyler and I have been joined by two other fly-fishing enthusiasts. Genie and Marion became "pros" with their fly-rods and were catching rainbows in Montana with the best of them!

BUFFALOES - 99   CANCER - 1
Gooo Buffaloes! We're doing it TEAM! I have just returned from Duke and a CAT scan. My doctor reports that the cancer continues to diminish and that I can count on Game 3 sometime in October. Game 2 was a tough one, and I feel I must tell you something because it's very important to the team concept.

In my quest for the Real Red Bike Jenny writes about in her letter, I became overzealous and ended up in Duke's intensive care unit again. When they wheeled me in, I was very, very weak. It was a difficult time, and I prayed for strength to get through the next couple of hours. I began thinking about my family, each of you, your calls, your letters and cards, the jokes, the books, the wonderful photographs you have sent and then I had the thought—Stone, you wimp! Suck it up, the Buffaloes are pulling for you and you need to get tough—I was out of there in a day and a half! My point is this—I could not have done it

139

without family and friends—the team concept works!

The other news I wish to share with you is that Genie and I have decided to move to the mountains. We had planned to retire there someday, but my medical situation has just moved it up a few years. It's sad to leave our friends in Greensboro, but we plan on keeping close ties and counting on you to come see us in the mountains.

I think that October 7th will be the day I return to Duke. If you have a chance, say a little prayer for us. It means so much. Genie, Tyler and Marion join me in sending you our love.

Love, Bob
"I always thank God for you..."
I Corinthians 1:4 NIV

140

September 7, 1990

YO, TEAM BUFFALO!

LATEST SCORE
BUFFALOES - 99.50 CANCER - 00.50

I heard from my doctor yesterday who had just compared my last two CAT scans, measuring how much the lesions on my lungs had diminished. Guess what, Gang? Of the six lesions that we have been tracking five are completely gone! We go back to Duke on September 30th to begin Game Three. Your support has made the difference so please keep up your thoughts and prayers for this next offensive push.

I think about the Real Red bike a great deal, and when OUR TEAM wins it, you can ride it anytime —squirrel tail handlebars and all!

Thanks again!

Love, Bob

WHERE THE BUFFALOES ROAM

November 22, 1990

Dear Team,

Happy Thanksgiving! The Stones have a great deal to be thankful for this year, and you are at the top of the list. Nine months ago when I asked you to take this journey with me, I had no idea that we would come from a score of Buffaloes 25 - Cancer 75 to our present tally of Buffaloes 99.5 - Cancer 00.50. This has been accomplished by the best medical care and knowledge and care available, an incredibly strong and supportive family, your thoughts and prayers, and a loving God who has answered them. I am one thankful guy to have family and friends like you.

Yogi Berra best summed up my last treatment at Duke when he said, "It was like deja vu all over again." I won't bother you with my "war story" but will simply say that my ole body could only take 11 of the 15 days of IL-2 treatment. We had hoped to get rid of the last remaining lesion on my right lung, but the CAT scan I had last week showed that it was still there. The good news is that it did not grow—we will continue to watch it on a monthly basis. In the meantime, Genie has me on a rigorous exercise program and a very nutritious diet. I feel good and my strength is coming back daily. We are extremely optimistic about the future.

Word from my cousin Jenny is that I am still in contention for the REAL RED bike which is still my main goal. With your continued support we'll win it!

142

Letters

The enclosed picture of the home team was made on our trip this summer out West. When you look at it know that Genie, Tyler, Marion and I love you and wish for you a very Merry Christmas and a joyous 1991!

Love, Bob

MEMO TO: *Tripp Winn*
             Schwinn Bicycle Company

FROM: *jsb*

IMPERATIVE YOU NOTIFY GIVERNY BLUE CROWD THAT THEY ARE OUT OF RED BIKE COMPETITION. OFFER REGRETS AND SMELLING SALTS. OUR HIGH PLAINS DRIFTER HAS CLEANED THEIR PLOW. KNOW IT. SUGGEST YOU REMOVE WHEEL CHOCKS AND READY MTB # REAL RED FOR SHIPMENT LATE OCTOBER.

HATE TO SAY IT BUT I TOLD YOU SO. HOW DO WE STAND ON SQUIRREL TAILS?

144

Christmas Day
December 25, 1990

FROM: Tripp Winn with Schwinn Bicycle
Company

CONGRATULATIONS, MR. BOB STONE!

*Our own independent audit has verified that you
are indeed the winner of The Schwinn Mountain
Bike Competition. While we were told to hold
MTB # REAL RED for January delivery we have
little control over the matter. A Red Bike is like a
divining rod. It will find a boy and his Christmas
in spite of carelessly thought-out schedules.
Every red bike we assemble knows exactly where
to go. We have observed this phenomenon time
and time again. Mr. Bob, can you just picture it!
Our Schwinn MTB # REAL RED, jaunty raccoon
tails flying, streaking down the highway, over hill
and hollow, dirt roads and gullied paths to find
its rightful place with you on this Christmas Day!
Ms. Stone-Humphries was right about one thing:
the Giverny blue bike would never have made it.*

*May the joy and peace of this season be with you
and yours. The SCHWINN COMPANY and the
undersigned sponsors wish you the merriest
Christmas ever.*

Happy Pedaling,

YOUR TWINS

JENNY HUMPHRIES
BETTY ROBINSON

YOUR POWER PRAYER WARRIORS

    DAVID GRIMES
    LARRY SITTON
    VIC COCHRAN

WITH SPECIAL THANKS TO TYLER STONE FOR LOGISTICAL SUPPORT AND TO ALL YOUR FAMILY AND FRIENDS FOR STEADFAST PRAYER SUPPORT.

Letters

March 1, 1991

Dear Team:

*1990 was the year of the Buffalo! The herd had
a starring role in Dances With Wolves; the
Buffalo Bills missed winning the Super Bowl by 3
feet; and our* TEAM - THE BUFFALOES *came on
strong in December and won the* REAL RED BIKE
*in a dramatic finish! Imagine my surprise on
Christmas morning when I received the enclosed
letter from Jenny, followed by Marion and Tyler
wheeling in my new red Schwinn. It was
wonderful!*

*When I wrote my first letter to you on March 16,
1990, I had cancer in my left kidney, my lymph
glands, my spleen, my liver, and both of my lungs.
The strange thing was that I looked good and felt
great for an ole dude just six weeks over fifty.
Today, I am just six weeks over fifty-one, look
good, feel great, and am tumor free! My last
scans were very positive. They show only one
small shadow on one lung—we can't tell if it's
scar tissue or the remains of a shrinking tumor.
How did this happen?*

*In my first letter I mentioned that my parents, my
grandparents, and my Sunday School teachers
taught me long ago that God is Love, and that I
was feeling this love in abundance through your
calls, letters, beautiful flowers and positive
thoughts. I am here today because of the love I
received from you, my family, and the wonderful
folks at Duke. Our bumper sticker reads*
BUFFALOES - UNDEFEATABLE CHAMPS. *We*

are a powerful team, and I thank GOD every day for you.

Norman Cousin's book, Head First: The Biology of Hope, *presents the rapidly mounting scientific evidence that hope, faith, love, will to live, purpose, laughter, and festivity can help combat serious illness. Most importantly, such attitudes can enhance the environment of medical treatment. Each of you has helped me with these attitudes. You are my heroes.*

As I did with my first letter, I am again asking the TEAM *to do the following things:*

1. Please read the following verses from the Bible that have meant so much to me:

Psalms 23:4	*Jeremiah 30:17*
John 6:47	*Psalms 31:24*
Proverbs 8:17	*John 3:16*
Isaiah 55:12	*I John 4:19*
Hebrews 11:1	*John 13:34,35*

2. Please read Head First: The Biology of Hope *by Norman Cousins and give a copy to someone in the medical community or to a friend who has been diagnosed with a serious illness.*

3. Call me if you or anyone you know gets cancer, and you think that I can help. I have met many brave and courageous people this year who have cancer and have given me hope. It is my desire to help anyone at any time. Give me a call.

4. If you haven't already, please send me your picture for the OFFICIAL TEAM PROGRAM. It represents the most powerful team on Earth.

5. My friends at the Duke Cancer Center would love your extra Girl Scout cookies. Send me your extra tickets to the Eastern Regionals!

6. Lastly, but most importantly, remember us in your prayers. You will always be in ours. Genie, Tyler, Marion and I love you very much.

Bob
Matthew 7:7,8

September 1, 1990

Yo, Mountain Buffalo,

Each day we await news from the world capitals: Washington, Paris, London, Baghdad, Amman, Riyahd and the Blue Ridge. I have a swap to propose for Buffalo negotiators—the oil price can go wherever, the Iraqis get out of Kuwait and C gets out of Buffalo territory, starting with an immediate withdrawal from all of the invaded areas. This will make red bicycles mandatory for all of us.

The reason for moving to the mountains is bureaucratic. The post office will not allow General Delivery mail after 30 days so you had to get a P.O. Box so you might as well move. I like it. The only logical conclusion to reach.

How about a film like The Bear? *Picture this:*

Scene I: A young buffalo is seen roaming the streets of an urban center. Young buffalo is constantly getting stung by bees, stepping on rattlesnakes, falling down cliffs and experiencing other travails because he repeatedly tries to live life to the fullest.

Scene II: A maturing but playful buffalo finds mate and begins family in new locale. Spends a lot of time hunting for the best place to graze, chasing other buffalos away, showing new buffalo calves where not to step and leading less fortunate wildlife to fresher water, greener grass and bluer skies.

150

Scene III: Buffalo watches as calves grow into buffaloes, too. Buffalo missus shows creative side. Green grass becomes harder to find, pressure rises to find fresh water, buffalo internalizes—bad for any buffalo. Suddenly, while buffalo internalizing, Indians (merely a metaphor, not a reflection on any ethic group) appear and buffalo catches a few arrows. Buffalo bellows. Other buffaloes circle wounded buffalo. Other wildlife, previously shown greener grass, fresher water, bluer skies by buffalo, return to circle around buffalo and drive Indians off. Buffalo nurses wounds. It is not easy but buffalo healing.

Scene IV: Buffalo stands on mountain top. Cool stream runs below. Water is fresh and plentiful. Grass has never been greener. Sky never bluer. Indians not a problem. Buffalo gets a post office box.

Your faith, determination and example offers us as much support as we offer you. You continue as a model for the efficient use of resources. You always put back more than you use. We think about you every day.

Love,
The Hazels

(Letter from Phil Hazel dated September 1, 1990)

Pam and I would like to act as attorney and agent when you write your memoirs. We think it has real appeal to the masses and we think we can get you a terrific deal with Touchstone Pictures. There has been some preliminary discussion in Hollywood on casting. It looks like Signourney Weaver is set for Genie, with either Tom Cruise in lifts or Alan Alda as the Buffalo. ...T-Shirts, coffee mugs and caps look to generate some real good cash flow. McDonalds is concepting a Buffalo-burger in test markets and they see it as a tie-in with Teenage Mutant Ninja IL-2 plus LAK. THE POSSIBILITIES ARE ENDLESS. Aaaahhh, but you already knew that.

(letter from Phil Hazel, not dated)

March 25, 1990

Dear Bob,

Your letters are fantastic and the weather reports delightful. I must add you to my creative "Think Tank." I should have known that you would make your "Journey" into a "Campaign."

Edward N. Booker, Jr.

(Letter from Edward N. Booker, Jr. dated March 25, 1990)

Letters

Tuesday, March 27, 1990

Buffalo,

*I couldn't resist taking this card along to
Tuesday Club this afternoon for all to sign. You
will note some signatures of people you never
heard of—I told them that didn't matter, that it
wouldn't upset you to know that a roomful of 30
women were all thinking about you, whether you
know them or not!*

*It was the usual hilarious meeting—Mrs.___went
sound asleep in the middle of the program, and
the hostess was sick in the bedroom with
bronchitis and never appeared. Jane was the co-
hostess in charge of refreshments but didn't know
it until yesterday but did an admirable job of
pulling Christmas fudge out of the freezer... You
know we're all behind you—and with the entire
Tuesday Club on your side, that is pretty
formidable.*

Love from all the Kimbroughs

(Letter from Tish Kimbrough dated 3-27-90)

October 7, 1991

Dear Bob:

*Thank you for taking control last Wednesday and
being an inspiration for Patty White. I did come
very near to breaking her arm to get her there so
you and the Lord could do the rest. (You and*

153

Genie did your part.) Since Wednesday night, she has changed so much. A real positive person. Changed from believing her doctor's gloom and doom report... Yesterday she called and asked if they could come show us their new toy. Five minutes later a 1966 GMC Coach arrived. They plan to convert it to a motor home.

Dan Kerns

(Letter from Dan Kerns dated October 7, 1990)

Dear Bob,

I've been wanting to write you for a long time but have never quite known how to start or what to say. The news of what has happened hit me very hard at first. For a couple of days I didn't know what to do or how to react. I was angry, hurt, mad, and sad—but then I finally began to think of how you must be reacting and what you would need from me and everyone else. It's not the tears or the sadness that are going to get us through this, but it's the support, the positive thinking, and the prayers.

(Letter from Jane Price dated September 3, 1990)

Letters

Dear Genie & Bob,

Since I returned to the U.S. November 14 (diagnosed with cancer) my whole life has changed in every conceivable way! I am learning many valuable lessons for living fully and with love and appreciation for the many, many friends who have supported me during this challenge.

Please continue to put out that positive energy through your thoughts, prayers and personal communication with me. Your cards, letters, pictures and calls will all help to keep me focused on the positive aspects of my treatment for the next six months. Remind me of the "good old times" I may have spent with you or particular episodes we have shared.

(Letter from Suzanne Lewis dated February 25, 1991)

Dear Genie & Bob,

Thank you both for taking me "under wing." I've read all the letters and articles over and over—what great family and friends to be on the "the team!!!" I would be proud to carry on with the Buffaloes down in Fort Lauderdale. I have several friends with cancer with whom I keep close contact, and if it's all right with the Buffaloes, I'd like to include them on the team.

(Letter from Mickie Andrews dated January 28, 1992)

Dear Children,

I have chosen you to adopt these bears. I found these poor things in a cave in Wyoming. I have wrapped them in plastic to keep them dry and warm. Take the plastic off when you get home and LOVE them!

Two things will be necessary to maintain their health. You must read some to them each day, and they love and adore Bach's Brandenburg concertos. You absolutely must get a record or tape and play Benjamin some each day. Hold his little paw and listen for 5 minutes, 3 times a week. It may sound strange to you at first but soon you will grow to love Bach as much as Benjamin does.

...Train your Teddy right. Read a little of your Bible or Torah to him each week, and give him lots and lots of bear hugs.

Sincerely, Ted D. Bear

(Letter from Martha Stone Woods, Bob's sister, to her first grade class, dated March 3, 1990)

Dear Bob,
We are So So
so sorry that your
sick! I know
someone that
has Cancer. Her
name is Susan
Jacobs. She is my
best friend. Bec-
ause she is very
nice

Love, Jim &
Imogene's your-
est daughter

Dear Bob
I hope ya like
the picture of me
that I gave ya.
It has somethi-
ng on the back
It say's that
I am Jim &
I am Imogene's youngest
daughter, and that
I'm 8 years old
Love Jim & Imoge-
ne's youngest daughter,
Rebecca

Sunday March 10, 1991

Dear Mrs. Woods First Grade,

You are my heroes!

You helped me get well with

Your letters and funny pictures.

You made me smile and

laugh which helped my

body's immune system attack

the cancer. Do you know

what happened? We kicked

the old cancer right out

of my body!

All of you are good

at writing letters, and they

help everyone you send them

to. Thank you for thinking

of me and helping me get

WELL! I Love you!!

Josh Stone

Mrs. Woods little brother

AFTERWORD

Bob Stone's story began with the wake-up call he got after a strenuous game of handball. That wake-up call parlayed itself into a team called the Buffaloes and a go-for-broke race for a Real Red bike outfitted with a pair of raccoon tails. Much happened in between.

As a writer of fiction, I was accustomed to moving people and predicaments across a blank page at will, devising my own solutions to life challenges. But writing about real life is more difficult. Bob couldn't do what I wanted him to do——say "Shazam!" like he did as a kid, and nuke his cancer with a salvo of thunderbolts. (Although Bob did try, give him that.)

Bob's answer to cancer was to put together a team. Bob talked about his team. He said we were his team. He even wrote to us and we wrote back. But does that make us a team or just good fiction?

I began to find out the answer as I watched Bob and Genie tell their story on *CBS This Morning*. Suddenly I saw that this was not just another cancer survivor's story. I had an exciting realization that many, many people felt connected to Bob and Genie Stone. Why, I asked myself? Was this his team?

I spent one very long night reading cards, letters, and cartoons which filled a duffle Bob dragged home from Duke. I was staggered by the breadth and depth of caring, from family, friends, doctors and others who cared for him—even from rank strangers. I became persuaded, then excited, that this outpouring was indisputable proof that we really were a team!

They convinced me that we all love to be a friend, in spite of friending being a very labor-intensive effort. Therein lies both the majesty and the mystery of the Buffaloes and all the other teams that come after. We all want to be a friend. We all want to help someone try. And we learn much in helping Bob try.

Jenny Stone Humphries

159

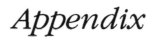

Appendix

THE NATIONAL CANCER INSTITUTE
CANCER CENTERS PROGRAM

The Cancer Centers Program is comprised of 57 NCI-designated Cancer Centers actively engaged in multidisciplinary research efforts to reduce cancer incidence, morbidity, and mortality. Within the program, there are four types of centers:

Basic Science Cancer Centers (15), which engage primarily in basic cancer research;

Clinical Cancer Centers (12), which focus on clinical research;

"Comprehensive" Cancer Centers (28), which emphasize a multidisciplinary approach to cancer research, patient care, and community outreach;

Consortium Cancer Centers (2), which specialize in cancer prevention and control research.

Although some cancer centers existed in the late 1960s and the 1970s, it was the National Cancer Act of 1971 that authorized the establishment of 15 new cancer centers, as well as continuing support for existing ones. The passage of the act also dramatically transformed the centers' structure and broadened the scope of their mission to include all aspects of basic, clinical, and cancer control research. Over the next two decades, the centers' program grew progressively.

In 1990, there were 19 comprehensive cancer centers in the nation. Today, there are 28 of these institutions, all of which meet specific NCI criteria for comprehensive status.

To attain recognition from the NCI as a comprehensive cancer center, an institution must pass rigorous peer review. Under guidelines newly established in 1990, the eight criteria for "comprehensiveness" include the requirement that a center have a strong core of basic laboratory research in several scientific fields, such as biology and molecular genetics, a strong program of clinical research, and an ability to transfer research findings into clinical practice.

Moreover, five of the criteria for comprehensive status go significantly beyond that required for attaining a Cancer Center Support Grant (also referred to as a P30 or core grant), the mechanism of choice for supporting the infrastructure of a cancer center's operations. These criteria encompass strong participation in NCI-designated high-priority clinical trials, significant levels of cancer prevention and control research, and important outreach and educational activities—all of which are funded by a variety of sources.

The other types of cancer centers also have special characteristics and capabilities for organizing new programs of research that can exploit important new findings or address timely research questions.

Of the 57 NCI-designated Cancer Centers, 15 are of the basic science type. These centers engage almost entirely in basic research, although some centers engage in collaborative research with outside clinical research investigators and in cooperative projects with industry to generate medical applications from new discoveries in the laboratory.

Clinical cancer centers, in contrast, focus on both basic research and clinical research within the same institutional framework, and frequently incorporate nearby affiliated clinical research institutions into their overall research programs. There are 12 such centers today.

Finally, consortium cancer centers, of which there are two, are uniquely structured and concentrate on clinical research and cancer prevention and control research. These centers interface with state and local public health departments for the purpose of achieving the transfer of effective prevention and control techniques from their research findings to those institutions responsible for implementing population-wide public health programs. Consortium centers are also heavily engaged in collaborations with institutions that conduct clinical trial research and coordinated community hospitals within a network of cooperating institutions in clinical trials.

Together, the 57 NCI-Designated Cancer Centers continue to work toward creating new and innovative approaches to cancer research and, through interdisciplinary efforts, to effectively move this research from the laboratory into clinical trials and into clinical practice.

Following is a list of the 57 NCI-designated Cancer Centers.

Comprehensive*, Clinical, and Consortium Cancer Centers
Supported by the National Cancer Institute**

Information about referral procedures, treatment costs, and services available to patients can be obtained from the individual cancer centers listed below.

ALABAMA

**University of Alabama at Birmingham
Comprehensive Center***
Basic Health Sciences Building, Room 108
1918 University Blvd.
Birmingham, AL 35294
Tel. (205) 934-6612

ARIZONA

University of Arizona Cancer Center*
1501 North Campbell Ave.
Tucson, AZ 85724
Tel. (602) 626-6372

CALIFORNIA

**The Kenneth T. Norris Jr.
Comprehensive Cancer Center***
University of Southern California
1441 Eastlake Ave.
Los Angeles, CA 90033-0804
Tel. (213) 226-2370

Jonsson Comprehensive Cancer Center*
University of California at Los Angeles
200 Medical Plaza
Los Angeles, CA 90027
Tel. (213) 206-0278

City of Hope National Medical Center**
Beckman Research Institute
1500 East Duarte Road
Duarte, CA 91010
Tel. (818) 359-8111, ext. 2292

University of California at San Diego Cancer Center**
225 Dickinson St.
San Diego, CA 92103
Tel. (619) 543-6178

COLORADO

University of Colorado Cancer Center**
4200 East 9th Ave., Box B190
Denver, CO 80262
Tel. (303) 270-7235

CONNECTICUT

Yale University Comprehensive Cancer Center*
333 Cedar St.
New Haven, CT 06510
Tel. (203) 785-6338

DISTRICT OF
COLUMBIA

Lombardi Cancer Research Center*
Georgetown University Medical Center
3800 Reservoir Rd. NW
Washington, DC 20007
Tel. (202) 687-2192

FLORIDA

Sylvester Comprehensive Cancer Center*
University of Miami Medical School
1475 Northwest 12th Ave.
Miami, FL 33136
Tel. (305) 548-4800

ILLINOIS

Illinois Cancer Center
17th Floor
200 South Michigan Ave.
Chicago, IL 60604
Tel. (312) 986-9980

University of Chicago Cancer Research Center**
5841 South Maryland Ave.
Chicago, IL 60637
Tel. (312) 702-9200

MARYLAND	**The Johns Hopkins Oncology Center*** 600 North Wolfe St. Baltimore, MD 21205 Tel. (301) 955-8638
MASSACHUSETTS	**Dana-Farber Cancer Institute*** 44 Binney St. Boston, MA 02115 Tel. (617) 732-3214
MICHIGAN	**Meyer L. Prentis Comprehensive Cancer Center** **of Metropolitan Detroit*** 110 East Warren Ave. Detroit, MI 48201 Tel.(313) 745-4329
	University of Michigan Cancer Center* 101 Simpson Drive Ann Arbor, MI 48109-0752 Tel. (313) 936-9583
MINNESOTA	**Mayo Comprehensive Cancer Center*** 200 First Street Southwest Rochester, MN 55905 Tel. (507) 284-3413
NEW HAMPSHIRE	**Norris Cotton Cancer Center*** Dartmouth-Hitchcock Medical Center 2 Maynard St. Hanover, NH 03756 Tel. (603) 646-5505
NEW YORK	**Memorial Sloan-Kettering Cancer Center*** 1275 York Avenue New York, NY 10021 Tel. 1-800-525-2225

Columbia University Comprehensive Cancer Center*
College of Physicians and Surgeons
630 West 168th St.
New York, NY 10032
Tel. (212) 305-6905

Roswell Park Cancer Institute*
Elm and Carlton St.
Buffalo, NY 14263
Tel. (716) 845-4400

Albert Einstein College of Medicine**
1300 Morris Park Avenue
Bronx, NY 10461
Tel. (212) 920-4826

Kaplan Cancer Center*
New York University Medical Center
462 First Avenue
New York, NY 10016-9103
Tel. (212) 263-6485

University of Rochester Cancer Center**
601 Elmwood Avenue, Box 704
Rochester, NY 14642
Tel. (716) 275-4911

NORTH CAROLINA   **Duke Comprehensive Cancer Center***
P. O. Box 3814
Durham, NC 27710
Tel. (919) 286-5515

UNC Lineberger Comprehensive Cancer Center*
University of North Carolina School of Medicine
Chapel Hill, NC 27599
Tel. (919) 966-4431

Cancer Center of Wake Forest University at the Bowman Gray School of Medicine*
300 South Hawthorne Road
Winston-Salem, NC 27103
Tel. (919) 748-4354

OHIO

Ohio State University Comprehensive Cancer Center*
410 West 10th Avenue
Columbus, OH 43210
Tel. (614) 293-8619

Ireland Cancer Center **
Case Western Reserve University
University Hospitals of Cleveland
2074 Abington Road
Cleveland, OH 44106
Tel. (216) 844-5432

PENNSYLVANIA

Fox Chase Cancer Center*
7701 Burholme Avenue
Philadelphia, PA 19111
Tel. (215) 728-2570

University of Pennsylvania Cancer Center*
3400 Spruce St.
Philadelphia, PA 19104
Tel. (215) 662-6364

Pittsburgh Cancer Institute*
200 Meyran Avenue
Pittsburgh, PA 15213-2592
Tel. 1-800-537-4063

RHODE ISLAND

Roger Williams Cancer Center**
825 Chalkstone Avenue
Providence, RI 02908
Tel. (401) 456-2071

TENNESSEE	**Drew-Meharry-Morehouse Consortium Cancer Center** 1005 D.B. Todd Blvd. Nashville, TN 37208 Tel. (615) 327-6927
	St. Jude Children's Research Hospital** 332 North Lauderdale St. Memphis, TN 38101-0318 Tel. (901) 522-0306
TEXAS	**Institute for Cancer Research and Care**** 4450 Medical Drive San Antonio, TX 78229 Tel. (512) 616-5580
	The University of Texas M.D. Anderson Cancer Center* 1515 Holcombe Blvd. Houston, TX 77030 Tel. (713) 792-3245
UTAH	**Utah Regional Cancer Center**** University of Utah Health Sciences Center 50 North Medical Drive, Room 2C10 Salt Lake City, UT 84132 Tel. (801) 581-5052
VERMONT	**Vermont Cancer Center*** University of Vermont 1 South Prospect St. Burlington, VT 05401 Tel. (802) 656-4580
VIRGINIA	**Massey Cancer Center**** Medical College of Virginia Virginia Commonwealth University 1200 East Broad St. Richmond, VA 23298 Tel. (804) 786-9641

WASHINGTON   **Fred Hutchinson Cancer Research Center***
                    1124 Columbia Street
                    Seattle, WA 98104
                    Tel. (206) 467-4675

WISCONSIN   **Wisconsin Clinical Cancer Center***
                    University of Wisconsin
                    600 Highland Avenue
                    Madison, WI 53792
                    Tel. (608) 263-8090

Basic Science Cancer Centers
Supported by the National Cancer Institute

La Jolla Cancer Research Foundation
La Jolla, CA

Armand Hammer Center for Cancer Biology, Salk Institute
San Diego, CA

Cancer Center, California Institute of Technology
Pasadena, CA

Purdue Cancer Center, Purdue University
West Lafayette, IN

The Jackson Laboratory
Bar Harbor, ME

Worcester Foundation for Experimental Biology
Shrewsbury, MA

Center for Cancer Research, Massachusetts Institute of Technology
Cambridge, MA

Eppley Institute, University of Nebraska Medical Center
Omaha, NE

Cold Spring Harbor Laboratory
Cold Spring Harbor, NY

Institute of Environmental Medicine
New York University Medical Center
New York, NY

American Health Foundation
New York, NY

Wistar Institute
Philadelphia, PA

Fels Research Institute, Temple University
School of Medicine
Philadelphia, PA

Cancer Center, University of Virginia
Health Sciences Center
Charlottesville, VA

McArdle Laboratory for Cancer Research
University of Wisconsin
Madison, WI

For additonal information about cancer, write:
Office of Cancer Communications
National Cancer Institute
Bethesda, MD 20892.

Or call the toll-free telephone number of the
Cancer Information service.
Spanish-speaking staff members are available.
1-800-4-CANCER

SELECTED BIBLIOGRAPHY

Anderson, Gary. *The Cancer Conqueror: An Incredible Journey to Wellness*. New York: Andrews & McMeel, 1990 (Paper).

Benjamin, Harold H. *From Victim to Victor*. New York: Dell, 1987.

Borysenko, Joan. *Minding the Body, Mending the Mind*. Reading: Addison-Wesley, 1987.

Brennan, Barbara Ann. *Hands of Light*. New York: Bantam, 1987.

Chopra, Deepak. *Quantum Healing*. New York: Bantam, 1989.

Cousins, Norman. *Anatomy of an Illness*. New York: Norton, 1979.

Cousins, Norman. *The Healing Heart*. New York: Norton, 1983.

Cousins, Norman. *Head First: The Biology of Hope*. New York: Dutton, 1989.

Frank, Arthur W. *At The Will of the Body: Reflections on Illness*. New York: Houghton-Mifflin, 1991.

Friedman, Howard. *The Self Healing Personality*. New York: Holt, 1991.

Hay, Louise L. *You Can Heal Your Life*. Santa Monica: Hay House, 1984.

Kronhausen, Eberhard and Phyllis with Demopolous, Harry B. *Formula for Life*. New York: William Morrow, 1989.

Marchetti, Albert. *Beating the Odds*. New York: St. Martin's Press, 1988.

Murphy, Joseph. *The Power of the Subconscious Mind.* New York: Prentice-Hall, 1963.

Nessim, Susan and Ellis, Judith. *Cancervive: The Challenge of Life After Cancer.* New York: Houghton-Mifflin, 1991.

Peck, M. Scott. *The Road Less Traveled.* New York: Simon & Schuster, 1987.

Roud, Paul. *Making Miracles.* New York: Warner, 1990.

Sattilaro, Anthony J. *Recalled By Life.* New York: Houghton-Mifflin, 1982.

Siegel, Bernie S. *Peace, Love and Healing.* New York: Harper & Row, 1989.

Siegel, Bernie S. *Love, Medicine and Miracles.* New York: Harper & Row, 1986.

Sher, Barbara and Gottlieb, Annie. *Teamworks.* New York: Warner, 1991.

Magazines

"American Health," RD Publications, 28 West 23rd St., New York, New York 10010.

"Coping," Pulse Publications, P.O. Box 1700, Franklin, TN 37065.

"Prevention Magazine," Rodale Press, 33 E. Minor St., Emmaus, PA 18049.

ABOUT THE AUTHORS

Bob Stone

Bob Stone grew up in Charlotte, North Carolina, the son of a Presbyterian minister. He graduated from Davidson College and is active in its alumni affairs. He has served on the Citizens Advisory Committee for the Duke Comprehensive Cancer Center. He is a committed, ardent worker for civic causes such as Child Care Ministry, Inc. Through the years, he and his wife, Genie, have taken seven foster children into their home to love. Bob is also an Elder in the First Presbyterian Church in Greensboro. Bob and Genie have two grown children, Marion and Tyler, and a not-so-grown golden retriever named Maggie. They now make their home in the Blue Ridge mountains of North Carolina, where Bob has a garden and talks daily by telephone with cancer patients world-wide. Bob is a much-in-demand speaker, telling the story of his team, which saw him through the biggest challenge of his life.

Bob is also an avid trail biker, and the only one riding a MTB # Real Red Schwinn, customized with genuine raccoon tails on the handlebars.

Jenny Stone Humphries

Jenny Stone Humphries was born and raised in Stoneville, North Carolina. After college, she worked for a large Atlanta advertising agency. Jenny and her husband Stan now live in Atlanta and have two adult children, Sally and Stanley Bradford.

Her short fiction has appeared in magazines and literary reviews, including the *North American Review*, the *Chariton Review*, and *The Greensboro Review*. Twice her stories were selected as Distinguished Stories of the Year in *The Best American Short Stories* and her fiction was cited in the *Pushcart Prize, XII*. *Where the Buffaloes Roam* is her first work of non-fiction. She is now at work on a book of family letters and continues to write fiction.

Jenny does not have a brother, but if she did, it would be Bob.